An Introduction to Evolutionary Cognitive Archaeology

An Introduction to Evolutionary Cognitive Archaeology is the first concise introduction that lays out the epistemological foundations of evolutionary cognitive archaeology in a way that is accessible to students.

The volume is divided into three sections. The first section situates cognitive archaeology in the pantheon of archaeological approaches and distinguishes between ideational cognitive archaeology and evolutionary cognitive archaeology. This is followed by a close look at the nature of cognitive archaeological inferences and concludes with brief summaries of the major methods of evolutionary cognitive archaeology. The second section of the book introduces the reader to a variety of cognitive phenomena that are accessible using the methods of cognitive archaeology: memory, technical cognition, spatial cognition, social cognition, art and aesthetics, and symbolism and language. The third section presents a brief outline of hominin cognitive evolution from the perspective of evolutionary cognitive archaeology. The authors divide the archaeological record into three major phases: The Bipedal Apes—3.3 million–1.7 million years ago; The Axe Age—1.7 million–300,000 years ago; and The Emergence of Modern Thinking—300,000–12,000 years ago.

An Introduction to Evolutionary Cognitive Archaeology is an essential text for undergraduate students, graduate students, and scholars across the behavioral and social sciences interested in learning about cognitive archaeology, including psychologists, philosophers, anthropologists, and archaeologists.

Thomas Wynn is a distinguished professor of anthropology at the University of Colorado, Colorado Springs. Since the 1970s, his research has centered on the explicit use of psychological theory to interpret archaeological remains. He has published extensively on hominin cognitive evolution.

Frederick L. Coolidge is a professor of psychology at the University of Colorado, Colorado Springs (UCCS). He is the co-director of the UCCS Center of Cognitive Archaeology. He is the author or co-author of several books spanning the disciplines of cognitive archaeology, statistics, and psychology.

An Introduction to Evolutionary Cognitive Archaeology

Thomas Wynn and
Frederick L. Coolidge

Routledge
Taylor & Francis Group
NEW YORK AND LONDON

Cover image: Dagmar Hollmann / Wikimedia Commons

First published 2022
by Routledge
605 Third Avenue, New York, NY 10158

and by Routledge
4 Park Square, Milton Park, Abingdon, Oxon, OX14 4RN

Routledge is an imprint of the Taylor & Francis Group, an informa business

Library of Congress Cataloging-in-Publication Data
A catalog record for this book has been requested

ISBN: 978-0-367-85695-3 (hbk)
ISBN: 978-0-367-85694-6 (pbk)
ISBN: 978-1-003-01448-5 (ebk)

DOI: 10.4324/9781003014485

Typeset in Goudy
by Apex CoVantage, LLC

Contents

Prologue

Evolutionary cognitive archaeology is a relatively new specialty in prehistoric archaeology, and there are few authoritative accounts of how it differs from other forms of archaeological enquiry. Our goal in the following short introduction is to present the methods of evolutionary cognitive archaeology as clearly as possible. We hope that readers will come away with an understanding of the distinct features of reasoning associated with the approach. We also provide a sample of some of the insights that evolutionary cognitive archaeology has provided to the understanding of human evolution. We presume that the reader has some familiarity with archaeological practice. We will bypass the nuts and bolts of field and laboratory work and jump directly to the nature of archaeological reasoning.

Section I

Method and Theory

1 Introduction

Archaeology is a set of methods for studying the past through analysis of the material remains of past activities. The oft-cited comparison to crime scene investigation is apt. Both analyze patterns of material things, mostly unintended by the original actors, and their environmental context. Most laypeople associate archaeology with the investigation of the deep prehistoric past—many even believe archaeologists study dinosaurs—but as a set of methods, archaeology is applicable to any past time frame including the present. Many academic disciplines rely on archaeology, including prehistory, history, art history, religious studies, and anthropology. Some of these disciplines claim to do scientific archaeology, but others make no such claims. Evolutionary cognitive archaeology (ECA) falls squarely on the scientific side of this divide.

Scientific archaeology is a historical science, similar in many respects to geology, paleontology, and physical geography. The historical sciences do not rely on experiments to provide data for interpretation. Instead, the historical sciences rely on observation and analysis of patterns generated by natural processes. The experimental sciences use experiments to test hypotheses about the natural world. Indeed, this is the archetypal model of scientific research—form a hypothesis, generate experiments that test predictions of the hypothesis, and assess the accuracy of the hypothesis based on the success or failure of the prediction (falsification). If historical sciences cannot formulate predictions that can be tested experimentally, how can they lay claim to scientific status? First, the historical sciences do form hypotheses and do test hypotheses through analysis of relevant data. They acquire the data through observation and measurement. In a sense, historical sciences also predict by predicting what future observations will reveal, predictions that can be falsified. Second, both experimental and historical sciences rely on the two essential components of all scientific thinking—analysis of evidence and interpretation using explicit ideas about how the phenomena of interest work. Science needs both. Data do not speak for themselves. They only make sense in light of a framework of ideas. In science, such a framework of ideas is a theory. Theories in science are not tentative guesses (hypotheses play that role) but are coherent explanations of natural phenomena. Some theories have been so well established that they are no longer under challenge (heliocentric solar system; evolution), others

DOI: 10.4324/9781003014485-2

are less certain and still under investigation (Darwinism; embodied cognition), and still others have been shown to be wrong or incomplete but are still useful (William Sheldon's body typing theory; Newtonian physics).

Evolutionary cognitive archaeology shares with most other branches of scientific archaeology an assumption that the past is knowable. From the perspective of the history and philosophy of science, this aligns ECA with the "realists," the set of scientists and philosophers who believe that science, when done properly, does in fact generate accurate descriptions of the universe we live in. The alternative stance, the antirealists, believes that science can only reach conclusions about whether or not data are consistent with theory, but that theories themselves are hopelessly encumbered by past experiences of the researchers and socio/cultural context, there being no fool-proof method for choosing among them. In other words, scientists see only what their theories allow them to see. This antirealist stance has had an important influence on archaeological practice. There are respected archaeologists who maintain that all our interpretations of the past are entirely culture bound and that every culture-bound story about the past is equally likely. ECA practitioners tend not to be quite so cynical and believe that with appropriate theories and data, it is in fact possible to learn something about the past, including the nature of past minds.

2 Evolutionary Cognitive Archaeology

How does ECA differ from other varieties of archaeology? At the level of data recovery, ECA is no different from other archaeologies. Practitioners rely on the same range of field and laboratory techniques that form the basis of all archaeological data recovery and for which archaeologists have acquired a very public image. Archaeological fieldwork is expensive, tedious, time consuming, often uncomfortable, and occasionally exciting. It is also governed by formal and informal ethical standards for thoroughness of recovery and observation, recording, preserving, and disseminating results. Indeed, the ethical constraints are such that many archaeologists devote most of their efforts to finding and describing archaeological remains. But this is only one step in archaeological reasoning (though it is the one that attracts students in the first place). Interpretations of remains require making inferences from these data to conclusions about the past. ECA differs from other archaeologies in the way it structures these inferences.

Sixty-five years ago, English archaeologist Christopher Hawkes (1954) published a characterization of archaeological interpretations that has come to be known as the "ladder of inference," though he himself did not label it as such. He proposed a ranking of inferences about the prehistoric past ordered by how easy it was to make sound inferences. For Hawkes, soundness required establishing links to well-documented phenomena in the present or the historically documented past. The easiest inferences, he suggested, concerned **techniques** for making and using artifacts. Still "fairly easy" are inferences about **subsistence economics**, which rely on analyses of food remains and information about the environment provided by natural scientists. "Considerably harder" are inferences about **sociopolitical institutions**, largely because the institutions themselves do not preserve (they are social phenomena) and because of equifinality—many different social systems produce nearly identical patterns of archaeological remains (Hawkes used size of huts as his example). Inferences about **religious institutions and spiritual life** are the most tenuous. Determining that remains are likely to have been religious is not the difficulty (Hawkes uses cave painting as his example). Interpreting the meaning is the challenge. Without being able to connect the remains to known, documented human societies, inferring meaning, according to Hawkes, is almost impossible.

DOI: 10.4324/9781003014485-3

Hawkes' basic idea is that prehistoric archaeologists have reliable access to a narrow range of prehistoric activities. This is why archaeologists have a lot to say about pots, stone tools, and what people ate, but relatively little to say about kinship systems and religion. His point was not that archaeologists should not try to document these things, only that it is extremely difficult. Much of what follows in this book concerns how one can make sound inferences about the nature of past minds. These inferences are not situated on the easy rungs of Hawkes' ladder. But they are also not the most tenuous. Indeed, in many instances cognitive inferences are a bit less tenuous than inferences about sociopolitical institutions.

Evolutionary cognitive archaeology focuses on the archaeological record of hominin evolution (hominin is short for *Hominini*, which is the biological taxon that includes *Homo sapiens*, earlier forms of *Homo*, and related bipedal apes such as *Australopithecus*). The time period of interest extended from the advent of stone tools over 3 million years ago to the present. The vast majority of this time (3.3 million to 12,000 years ago) falls in the Palaeolithic, or Old Stone Age, as defined by archaeologists. The Palaeolithic was an immense span of time, and its sheer magnitude requires archaeologists of the Palaeolithic to adopt an evolutionary frame of reference, as opposed to the historic/modern frame of reference used by most archaeologists. When working within the historic/modern frame, archaeologists are able to recognize groups of people, even at social scales above the level of residential groups, and trace their development and fate on familiar landscapes. Archaeologists within this reference frame simply assume that their prehistoric and more recent actors possessed all the talents and abilities of modern humans. Archaeologists of the Palaeolithic do not have this luxury. Indeed, tracing the development of modern abilities is one of the primary goals of Palaeolithic archaeology. The differing frames of reference carry other methodological consequences. The evolutionary frame has a sliding scale of resolution. The further back in time a Palaeolithic archaeologist looks, the less there remains to see, a result of the chemistry of preservation, the ravages of erosion and other natural processes, and the smaller number of original actors on the landscape. Establishing chronology is always a challenge. Prehistoric archaeologists working in the modern/historic frame are often able to date their sites and artifacts very precisely, even to exact years in certain unusual cases. Archaeologists of the Palaeolithic are rarely able to date sites to a precise millennium and often treat sites separated by thousands of years as if they were the same age. One consequence of this lower level of chronological resolution is that the third rung of Hawkes' ladder—inferences about sociopolitical institutions—is especially difficult to study. At best, Palaeolithic specialists see single residential groups at a single point in time. This group's membership in or links to other groups are difficult to see. Thus, Palaeolithic specialists, including ECA practitioners, are effectively limited to analyzing individual actors, residential groups, and large-scale evolutionary trends.

Analysis at an evolutionary scale requires familiarity with evolutionary patterns and processes, both microevolution (one generation to the next) and macroevolution (hundreds of generations). ECA practitioners must understand how evolutionary change occurs, both biologically and culturally. Of particular relevance are processes of brain evolution, and also coevolutionary models of culture change such as niche construction theory, the ratchet effect, genetic assimilation, and neural reuse. These bodies of knowledge are not particularly onerous to acquire, but they are quite different from the patterns and processes encountered at the historic/modern frame of reference.

Evolutionary cognitive archaeology draws its most important ideas from cognitive science, and this is arguably the single most distinctive feature of the approach. As mentioned earlier, scientific reasoning requires evaluation of evidence (data) in the context of a set of ideas about how the natural world works (theory). Most Palaeolithic archaeologists rely on theories developed in the biological sciences, with **behavioral ecology** being arguably the most popular. Behavioral ecology, as the label itself indicates, is a set of well-developed ideas about how behavior enhances the survival and reproductive success of an organism in its ecological setting. Diet, foraging techniques and patterns, group size and organization, and life history patterns are some of the important foci of the approach. It is popular in Palaeolithic studies because many of the important variables are visible in the archaeological record (e.g., diet from refuse, foraging techniques from analysis of tools). But behavioral ecology has only a tangential interest in cognition, treating it primarily as a unitary phenomenon reflected in brain size and selected by other components of the theory (e.g., fruit eating primates have larger brains than leaf eating primates because of the challenge of finding ripe fruit). Thus, if one is interested in the evolution of cognition, behavioral ecology provides only a limited set of useful ideas.

Theory is well developed in the cognitive sciences and is based on 150 years of research. Indeed, the challenge for ECA is not the availability of appropriate theory but choosing among alternative, well-established theories of mental life. For example, the study of child development has inspired several theories of cognitive functioning, and because change is a critical component of these theories, they seemed a natural fit for evolutionary studies. Some of the earliest serious attempts at ECA grounded their interpretation in Jean Piaget's theory of cognitive development (Parker & Gibson, 1979; Piaget, 1970; Wynn, 1979). Although this approach provided a few lasting insights, it ultimately failed as a comprehensive theory, and the reasons are informative. First, ontogeny (sequence of individual development) and phylogeny (evolutionary development) do not share processes of change; indeed, Piaget's proposed mechanism was arguably non-Darwinian. Second, predictions drawn from the theory about the probable sequence of evolutionary change were falsified by the archaeological record itself. Failure of Piaget's model does not, of course, vitiate all models drawn from developmental psychology. More recently, Mark Moore has made effective use of a model of early ontogenetic change proposed by Patricia Greenfield (Greenfield, 1991; Moore, 2011).

Evolutionary cognitive archaeologists currently rely on a variety of models drawn from cognitive science. The most popular is **cognitive neuroscience**, which is an ambitious theory of brain function and cognition based on the experimental research of cognitive psychology and the brain function research of neuropsychology and neural imaging. A good example is neuroaesthetics. Experimental psychologists (Leder et al., 2004; Leder & Nadal, 2014) have identified several distinct cognitive components involved in aesthetic experience, and neuroscientists have been able to describe the neural networks that enable each of them (Chatterjee, 2014). The result is a powerful theory that archaeologists have used to understand the evolution of art (Berlant & Wynn, 2018; Hodgson, 2000), including the important conclusion that hominins made aesthetic evaluations long before there is any evidence for symbolic meaning (Wynn & Berlant, 2019).

A few more words about scientific theories are in order. To repeat, theories are the sets of ideas that scientists use to make sense of their data. One cannot make interpretations without a theory, and it is better to be explicit about the theory underpinning one's interpretations than not. Even commonsense expectations about the nature of reality are in fact underpinned by sets of ideas. One such commonsense expectation in archaeology is that throughout the past, events followed one another in a sequential fashion. This is a theory about the nature of time, and it is technically false, having been superseded in physics by space-time. It is even questionable from the perspective of folk theories of time. In Mesoamerica, for example, people thought of time as consisting of repeating cycles of events, not a linear sequence. The point is merely this—even our commonsense understandings are grounded in theory. Explicit, scientific theories vary a great deal in their scope and their power to explain. Scientists do think about large-scale theories of everything, modern big bang cosmology being an excellent example, but more often scientific theories focus on smaller problems. "Evolution," for example, is a theory about the nature and history of life. "Working memory," on the other hand, is a theory about the nature of executive thinking. It was proposed 45 years ago by Alan Baddeley and Graham Hitch (Baddeley & Hitch, 1974). The theory has been very successful in explaining certain aspects of mental life and has guided thousands of research projects, including research into the evolution of the human mind itself (Coolidge & Wynn, 2005; Wynn & Coolidge, 2010b). Students often complain when required to learn theory, as if it were somehow secondary to the facts of their chosen field of study. But without theory, there would be no facts, just meaningless heaps of data. Because ECA is a comparatively new academic specialty, its practitioners are often very careful to situate their reasoning within the limits of an explicit theory, but not always.

Outcomes

What does the knowledge generated by ECA look like? Another way to phrase this question would be to ask what we want to know from ECA. This is not a frivolous question, and it has important consequences for the future of the approach. Like most archaeology, practitioners use ECA to describe sequences of development over time and/or describe individual points in time in as much detail as possible. Traditionally, Palaeolithic specialists have always done both, as when they describe a sequence of technological phases or stages (e.g., Aurignacian, Solutrean, Magdalenian) or describe the daily life of people who lived at Dolni Vestonice-Pavlov 30,000 years ago (Svoboda, 2020). The result is a kind of narrative of hominin prehistory spanning three million plus years. ECA can enhance this standard narrative by providing information about the cognitive abilities of the protagonists. A good example of this is our book *How to Think Like a Neandertal* (Wynn & Coolidge, 2012), in which we tried to describe the cognitive life world of Neandertals and contrast it with that of modern humans. In this approach, ECA practitioners follow the lead of general paleoanthropology and provide insights into the hominin evolutionary narrative. They rely on paleoanthropology to provide the story line.

There is another way to frame the results of ECA. Instead of relying on paleoanthropology for a framework, turn to cognitive science itself. It is possible, for example, to focus on specific cognitive abilities and describe how they have evolved. Wynn (Wynn, 1979, 1989, 2002) and Hodgson (Hodgson, 2000, 2009, 2015) have done this for spatial cognition and have been able to demonstrate that modern abilities in spatial thinking, including the ability to imagine scenes from a variety of shifting points of view, had evolved by 500,000 years ago, long before anatomically modern humans had appeared on the scene. This approach is likely to be far more interesting to cognitive science in general, where its results articulate directly with cognitive neuroscience and evolutionary psychology. ECA can also compile the results for several different cognitive abilities and produce a parallel narrative to the traditional one used in paleoanthropology. At the end of this volume, we will provide an example of how this might look.

Research

What does one's research look like if one is a specialist in ECA? Many ECA specialists run field research projects using site survey and excavation techniques. This is nuts-and-bolts archaeology, no different from the fieldwork performed by other archaeologists. True, ECA may influence choice of geographic location and choice of sites, but in truth, serendipity and archaeological ethics are major determinants as well. One cannot simply study the bits one finds interesting; archaeological ethics require as exhaustive a documentation as possible, given time and financial constraints. It is after completion of fieldwork and basic description that ECA comes into play. Fieldwork is not the only source of data. The museums of the world are stuffed with millions and millions of artifacts, most of which have received only cursory description, if that. The romance of archaeology is in the field, not the museum dungeon, and even famous archaeological sites remain underreported. (The tomb of Egypt's King Tutankhamen, perhaps the most famous archaeological site of all, has never been formally described and published!) Thousands of potential PhD projects lie gathering dust. Thus, studying museum collections is a major avenue for ECA research.

Experimental research is also a component of ECA, primarily to investigate the cognitive underpinnings of activities, such as stone knapping, that are common in the archaeological record, but which have received no attention in experimental psychology. When doing this kind of experimental work, ECA specialists often team with experimental psychologists and neuroscientists and publish the results in both archaeological and neuroscience venues. Thus, ECA is truly interdisciplinary and multidisciplinary. Several current ECA practitioners specialize in this kind of research (Morgan et al., 2015; Putt et al., 2014; Stout et al., 2015).

Evolutionary cognitive archaeologists also rely on the efforts of other archaeologists. Archaeological ethics require public dissemination of results, and descriptions of evidence found by others is important to all archaeological interpretations. But other archaeologists may describe the data in ways that are not optimal for ECA. In these cases, it is necessary to redescribe the evidence, after first asking permission (professional courtesy) from the original researcher and the institution curating the evidence.

3 Two Cognitive Archaeologies

Two groups of scholars lay claim to the label "cognitive archaeology"—evolutionary cognitive archaeologists (ECA) and, for want of a better term, "ideational cognitive archaeologists" (ICA). They have separate histories and separate epistemologies. ICA has roots in historical archaeology and iconography and has occasionally embraced the theoretical stances of antirealist epistemology. ECA has roots in paleoanthropology and cognitive neuroscience and relies largely on realist scientific epistemology (Abramiuk, 2012). However, both share a commitment to understanding the role of human mindedness in the past and an antipathy to narrow materialist explanations. The groups are not mutually exclusive, but the differences in epistemology and topics of study mean that few scholars pursue both lines of research. The differences also make writing a comprehensive, but short, introduction almost impossible.

Ideational Cognitive Archaeology

Ideational cognitive archaeologists are interested in the content of past minds and in how mental phenomena, especially ideas, directed human action. The focus of ICA is on the recent past and on historic and prehistoric groups for whom it is possible to trace a direct link to people living today. Such links open up possibilities for discovering the meaning of symbols and other semiotically loaded phenomena (recall Hawkes' emphasis on these links in his ladder of inference). An excellent example is David Whitley's (2008) study of rock art in the Coso Mountains of the Mojave Desert in California, USA. There, Native Americans produced over 10,000 petroglyphs, which they engraved into basalt canyon walls. Images include stylized humans, desert bighorn sheep, and geometric designs. Archaeologists have identified several repetitive motifs, and Whitley interpreted these motifs using interviews with living descendent communities and ethnographic accounts written in the nineteenth century and early twentieth century. He was able to identify a powerful "conceptual metaphor" in the art, which he labeled KILLING A BIGHORN. Because his analysis was informed by ethnographic accounts, he knew that this metaphor did not address hunting, but instead referenced shamans passing into a trance state. Moreover, because petroglyphs have a time depth in the Great Basin of almost

DOI: 10.4324/9781003014485-4

11,000 years, Whitley was able to argue for a long period of cultural and symbolic continuity. Whitley's analysis differs from our account of the Hohlenstein-Stadel figurine (see pages 15–17). Whitley is concerned with *what* the motifs meant to the people who made them. We are content to identify *that* such meanings were likely to have been in play. Also, the routes to their respective conclusions were quite different. Whitley grounded his analysis in cognitive anthropology, theories of metaphor in particular (Lakoff & Johnson, 1980, 1999), which is in keeping with the semiotic/meaning orientation of ICA in general.

Because ICA analyses rely heavily on established links to living people, the weight of its conclusions attenuates the farther back in time one looks. The earliest focus of ICA interpretations are attempts to decipher Upper Palaeolithic cave art and figurines, but the results have been comparatively weak. It is impossible to link the artists to known groups of living people, beyond a too-general link to modern humans in Western Eurasia.

Although no one has ever made a count, it is almost certain that ICA practitioners outnumber those of ECA, a reflection of the comparatively fewer archaeologists who study human evolution.

Evolutionary Cognitive Archaeology

Evolutionary cognitive archaeologists study the evolution of specified and well-defined cognitive abilities. They are not, of course, the only scholars studying these phenomena. ***Paleoneurologists*** study the fossil evidence of brain evolution using a variety of techniques for measuring brain size and brain shape (Bruner, 2004, 2015). They identify evolutionary changes in the gross anatomy of the brain, including changes in relative proportions of major structures. Changes in brain size and shape certainly imply changes in brain function as well, but at neuroscience's current level of understanding, it is not yet possible to identify specific cognitive changes from brains alone. ***Evolutionary psychologists*** also study cognitive evolution but are primarily concerned with how cognitive abilities help people solve adaptive problems (Dunbar et al., 2005). They are less interested in the actual sequence of development (more on evolutionary psychology later). ***Comparative psychologists*** are a third group of scholars who study the evolution of brains and cognition (Tomasello & Herrmann, 2010). They focus on nonhumans and provide useful insights into brain evolution in general that are also relevant to understanding human evolution. Finally, ***primatologists*** study nonhuman primates, and many primatologists are interested in cognitive evolution (Matsuzawa et al., 2011).

ECA grounds itself in evolutionary theory and cognitive science. ECA has a macroevolutionary focus, emphasizing long-term evolutionary changes that occurred over the course of thousands of generations, rather than the microevolutionary processes that change populations over the short term. Thus, in addition to standard Darwinian models, ECA also invokes non-Darwinian patterns and processes such as genetic drift, the Baldwin effect (Weber & Depew, 2003), gene-culture coevolution, and neuronal reuse models (Dehaene &

Cohen, 2007). The primary focus of ECA is on what occurred in hominin cognitive evolution and the sequence of development. ECA grants priority to the archaeological record of change and treats the paleoneurological evidence of brain evolution as a parallel macroevolutionary sequence. One of the current puzzles of hominin cognitive evolution is the low level of concordance between these two records. Changes in hominin brains occurred without clear changes in the archaeological record, and significant developments in cognition occurred without apparent change in brain size and shape.

ECA is also grounded in cognitive science; it is this feature that provides its interpretive power. Rather than rely on commonsense notions of mental function, ECA turns to scientific theories of cognition, primarily those developed in the psychological sciences. Psychology is a vast field of study that subsumes many different approaches to human mental phenomena. (The American Psychological Association currently recognizes 45 major subdivisions.) The psychological sciences are distinguished by their adherence to scientific method and by their use of experimentation and statistical analysis. This results in descriptions of cognitive phenomena that have predictive power, and that are susceptible to further test and evaluation, that is, a set of descriptions that archaeologists can apply to their peculiar set of data. There is one dark spot to this otherwise friendly picture. Experimental psychology almost never directly tests the kinds of activities that produced the archaeological record in the first place. Tools and garbage are the bread and butter of prehistoric archaeology, but the activities responsible are complex, messy, and difficult to control in experimental protocols. However, experiments can focus on components of complex activities. It is then one of the tasks of the cognitive archaeologist to specify how these components impact the archaeological record itself (much more on this later).

Evolutionary Psychology

Novice students unfamiliar with academic labels often confuse ECA with evolutionary psychology (EP); the two labels are certainly similar. But the approaches to cognitive evolution are more different than the labels suggest, and it is important for an introductory text such as this to be clear about the distinction.

Evolutionary psychology is a variety of experimental psychology that strives to account for psychological phenomena in evolutionary terms. However, it is not primarily concerned with the evolutionary past per se. Instead, it focuses on how psychological phenomena function as adaptive mechanisms. Famously, for example, David Buss et al. (2003) argued the human males have a perceptual preference for women with a waist-to-hip ratio of about 80% (regardless of BMI) because this ratio is typical of young women with high potential fertility (fecundity); thus, the male perceptual bias is an *adaptation* for identifying fecund females. EP is narrowly Darwinian in its theoretical stance. It considers individual reproductive success (natural selection) to be the primary force in evolutionary change, though it does grant importance to kin selection as well, especially for psychological traits such as altruism that do not maximize individual success. EP is unusual among the evolutionary sciences in its reliance on reverse engineering as a research method. If a psychological phenomenon appears to be well-designed to solve a particular evolutionary problem (e.g., finding a mate), then it is probable that natural selection has engineered the result. EP practitioners rely on experiments to identify examples of good design, primarily experiments using human subjects, but occasionally using nonhuman primates to provide evolutionary context. EPs show little interest in the paleoanthropological record, preferring instead to rely on a hypothetical context based on knowledge of modern hunters and gatherers known as the Environment of Evolutionary Adaptedness (EEA). Modern psychological phenomena are thus understood as adaptations to the EEA, not modern urban life.

The evolution of spatial cognition illustrates the distinction between EP and ECA. In the 1990s, evolutionary psychologist Irwin Silverman et al. (2000, 2007) investigated the well-known but poorly understood sex difference in spatial cognition using a series of experiments, including experiments in wayfinding, which is one's ability to navigate landscapes intuitively without assistance of gadgets such as GPS and compasses. They found that young men typically outperformed young women, even when they controlled for experience. In paper-and-pencil tests, they found that males had an advantage in mental rotation, which is based on one's ability to imagine alternative visual points of view (allocentric perception is the formal term). They concluded that the male advantage in allocentric perception resulted from natural selection for males who could wayfind effectively while hunting, especially when required to navigate novel routes. Women also had a spatial advantage in identifying the location of multiple objects in complex backgrounds, an adaptation for gathering. Thus, the sex difference in spatial cognition is a good design for hunter-gatherers with a gender difference in foraging. At about the same time, archaeologists Thomas Wynn (1989, 2002) and Derek Hodgson (2006, 2015) studied the evolution of the spatial cognition used in stone tool manufacture. They demonstrated that spatial abilities in allocentric perception were in evidence by at least 500,000 years ago and probably much earlier. This was long before archaeological evidence for modern hunting and gathering with a gendered division of labor. Note that this archaeological conclusion does not disprove the EP interpretation of allocentric perception as being good evolutionary design, but it does falsify the hypothesis about the specific selective agent.

ECA and EP are not inherently contradictory, and indeed, research into the Social Brain Hypothesis (Dunbar, 1993; Dunbar et al., 2014) strove to integrate both. Robin Dunbar initially proposed the hypothesis to explain a provocative correlation between primate social group size and the size of primate neocortices and expanded it to be an EP hypothesis about social complexity selecting for specific cognitive abilities, including "Theory of Mind". Dunbar et al. then turned to the paleoanthropology and ECA to provide tangible evidence from the human fossil and archaeological records (Dunbar et al., 2014).

4 Reasoning About Prehistoric Minds

All archaeologists infer past activities from material remains; this is the essence of archaeological reasoning. But do material remains preserve anything of the minds of past actors? The facile answer is "of course, we all make inferences about minds based on material evidence." When looking at a house we decide whether the builder made a clever use of space or not. Similarly, when we observe a work of art we access the mind of the artist, unmediated by words and language. In other words, we regularly make commonsense evaluations based on material evidence. Psychology takes such evaluations a step further by situating them within the context of psychological theories. Neuropsychologists often ask patients with suspected brain trauma to draw a scene or a clock face. Individuals with some forms of brain damage produce distorted drawings (e.g., as when individuals suffering lateral neglect cluster all the numbers on one side of the clock face), and neuropsychologists use this physical evidence in their diagnoses. Developmental psychologists often ask children to draw, and indeed, there is an interesting and robust literature on the developmental implications of different kinds of drawn figures (Golomb, 1992; Kellogg, 1969).

Archaeologists can also make inferences about minds from material remains. Consider for a moment the Hohlenstein-Stadel figurine:

About 40,000 years ago, an ice age hunter-gatherer living in what is today Germany carved this figurine out of a piece of mammoth tusk (Conard, 2003). It is 28 cm in height. Even from a commonsense perspective, this artifact is a provocative window into a prehistoric mind. The creature depicted is not of this world, or even of the German Ice Age. It has a human body and a lion head; the term for such Frankenstein creatures is therianthrope. It is an imaginary creature; someone had to think it into existence. Perhaps, the maker saw the creature in a dream, or more likely produced it as an intentional act of creation. It strikes most people who see it as an example of religious iconography, that is, an image of a supernatural being. Such an interpretation relies on one's experience in the modern world where such images often play that role. The mind that thought this artifact is thus familiar to us.

A cognitive archaeological interpretation of the therianthrope differs from a commonsense interpretation by its explicit use of theory. In 2009, we teamed with one of our students to evaluate the Hohlenstein-Stadel figurine using

DOI: 10.4324/9781003014485-5

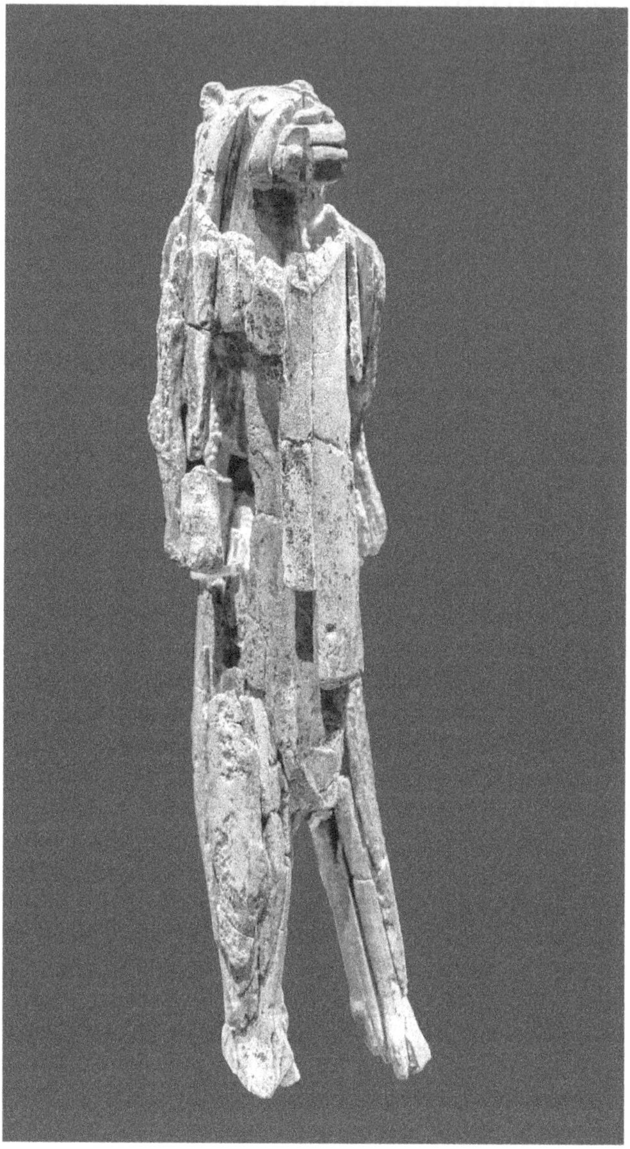

Figure 1 Hohlenstein-Stadel therianthrope, ca. 28 cm. Dagmar Hollmann/Wikimedia Commons. License: CC BY-SA 4.0.

concepts drawn from cognitive neuroscience (Wynn et al., 2009). We concluded that the artisan used varieties of conceptual thought, including a folk taxonomy of life forms, and that the melding of features from different conceptual domains required abstract thinking enabled by modern working memory capacity. Note that we made no attempt to discover what the therianthrope "meant" in a symbolic or religious sense. Instead, we focused on underlying cognitive mechanisms that were necessary for such an act of creation and were able to identify why the artisan was entirely modern in a cognitive sense.

In this analysis of Hohlenstein-Stadel, the artifact preserved something of the mind that thought it, and archaeologists interpreted the pattern. But artifacts can also play an active role in thinking, a role that was important in cognitive evolution itself. Smartphones make us smarter—able to solve problems we otherwise could not solve. So can an abacus, but it is much, much older. Indeed, the idea of number itself appears to have arisen through hominin engagement with artifacts as problem-solving devices (Overmann, 2013). Overmann argues that prehistoric people developed the concept of cardinal numbers gradually over the course of thousands of years through manipulation of fingers and material objects such as beads and iconic tokens. More interesting for us, some of this sequence is preserved in the archaeological record, documenting a form of coevolution of material culture and brains.

In the 1960s and early 1970s, academic archaeology passed through a period of intellectual turmoil concerning its basic approach to understanding the past (Hawkes' ladder of inference paper was a precursor to this debate). Part of the turmoil concerned archaeology's status as a science, which in post-WWII academia had skyrocketed in intellectual esteem. Many archaeologists disdained the notion that they were scientists, but others, especially North American prehistoric archaeologists, came to see this as the only viable approach to understanding and to any claim to relevance in the nonacademic world. At the heart of this disagreement was the basic epistemological question of whether archaeologists could or should reason scientifically. At the time, the Vienna School was still very influential in the philosophy of science [though on the wane, as exemplified by Thomas Kuhn's very influential *Structure of Scientific Revolutions* (Kuhn, 1962)] and its version of scientific reasoning became the model of scientific reasoning embraced by the "New Archaeology." The Vienna School championed deductive reasoning as the only path to scientific explanation. In deductive reasoning, one formulates a hypothesis and then uses it to generate predictions about the results of test cases, typically experiments of some kind. If predictions fail, the hypothesis is falsified. A requirement for all scientific hypotheses is that they must be susceptible to falsification. If the prediction is successful, the hypothesis is supported, but not proven. In strict deduction, hypotheses cannot logically be proven, only disproven, a logical quirk that eventually led to the abandonment of deduction as the sole arbiter of scientific explanations. Nevertheless, zealots of the New Archaeology strove to present their research in these hypothetico-deductive terms. The results were, as you might guess, often rather awkwardly constructed interpretations. After all, archaeology is not an experimental science.

Today, few archaeologists lay out their interpretations in the form of narrowly deductive arguments, but the New Archaeology (not so new anymore!) did succeed in establishing scientific reasoning as a baseline component of epistemology for many, but certainly not all, archaeologists. Instead of adherence to strict hypothetico-deductive reasoning, modern scientific archaeology, including ECA, embraces a more general commitment to sound reasoning that includes both inductive and deductive elements, reliance on explicit use of theory, and the careful marshalling of relevant archaeological data. ECA has its own set of challenges linked primarily to the necessity of connecting archaeological data to scientific understandings of the mind. Most practitioners rarely "step out" of their interpretive context to address the organizational structure of ECA reasoning in general. Two who have are Thomas Wynn and Rudolf Botha.

Wynn and Coolidge's Stipulations

In 2009, Wynn and Coolidge laid out the framework of reasoning that had guided Wynn's research for over 30 years, and which they believed provided a good standard for constructing persuasive interpretations in ECA (Wynn & Coolidge, 2009). ECA research, they suggested, must have both psychological and archaeological validity, and this validity has three components:

(1) **The cognitive ability under investigation must be recognized and defined by cognitive science; commonsense terms are not suitable.** All psychological approaches, including the psychological sciences, are plagued by a perennial problem. Most people think that they know how the mind works; after all, they have minds and use them introspectively to make general assertions about mindedness. Such introspection, along with culturally learned terms and understandings, constitutes a "folk psychology" that people use in their daily lives to negotiate their interactions with other people. It provides them with a practical utility that reinforces the reality of their folk terms. Early in the history of psychological research, psychologists realized that introspection was a poor research strategy and that folk psychology yielded results that were often just plain wrong. Unfortunately, some of these folk terms seem scientific and become the focus of commonsense approaches to cognitive archaeology. "Forward planning" and "symbolic thought" are two such terms. It is not that psychology has no interest in planning and symbolism. They are just not valid psychological constructs. Instead, psychologists rely on alternative, well-defined and circumscribed abilities identified through experimental research. For an ECA interpretation to be persuasive, it must use concepts and terms whose validity has been established through well-controlled research protocols.

(2) **The activities identified through archaeological evidence must have required the cognitive ability under investigation.** If another, simpler, cognitive ability could have organized the activity, it must be granted priority. Wynn initially labeled this stipulation "minimum necessary competence," but it is in fact simply a reformulation of logical parsimony. For example, one could argue that the bilateral symmetry evident on 1.7-million-year-old stone tools provides evidence for a Euclidean understanding of space, with three-dimensionality and allocentric (viewpoint

independent) perception. But, in fact, the minimum necessary competence is a perceptual preference for balance in the visual field, which does not require the more sophisticated abilities of Euclidean thinking.

(3) **The archaeological remains must have required the posited activity for which cognitive significance has been claimed.** Many archaeological patterns are subject to "equifinality." Often, different activities produce similar, even identical, archaeological signatures. This is yet another application of logical parsimony, this time on the archaeological evidence. A classic archaeological debate, still unresolved after 50 years, concerns the remains of butchered animals at the FLK 22 site at Olduvai Gorge (ca. 1.8 Ma). There are thousands of fragmentary animal bones, some with cutmarks produced by stone tools. Is this evidence for hunting or scavenging, a difference that caries potential cognitive implications? The default position in ECA must be that it represents scavenging, as this is the simpler strategy from a cognitive perspective.

These three stipulations have some practical consequences for ECA research that some archaeologists find onerous. An ECA researcher is as much a cognitive scientist as an archaeologist. One must not only know the terms and concepts of cognitive science but also understand the research milieu that proposed them. Unfortunately, few university programs in archaeology require students to obtain the necessary background in cognitive science. Of course, the reverse is true. Psychology programs rarely, if ever, require students to take courses in human evolution, let alone archaeology. This may explain the popularity of evolutionary psychology as a research approach in cognitive evolution; students who are never exposed to archaeology are unlikely to appreciate its potential.

Wynn and Coolidge's stipulations are general guidelines for ECA reasoning. Botha's model of reasoning provides a more detailed, and thus more powerful, account of the logic of ECA reasoning. He developed the model, which he labels the "windows approach," to address inadequacies in arguments about the evolution of language, but its structure can be applied directly to any scientific reasoning about the past (Botha, 2016, 2020).

Botha's Windows

Botha focuses on the construction of sound inferences, an inference being any conclusion based on evidence and reasoning. ECA reasoning consists of chains of inferences, and each of the links in a chain must be sound for the overall conclusion to be sound. Fig. 2 presents the chain of inference that we used in our interpretation of the Hohlenstein-Stadel figurine.

In the initial link of this inferential chain (ABC), content in the left "window" (A) consists of relevant data, content in the right window (C) is the conclusion, and the arrow connecting them is the inference (B). The data (A) are all features of the artifact; the conclusion (C) is that the artifact represents an imaginary beast that its makers could never have observed. For the inference

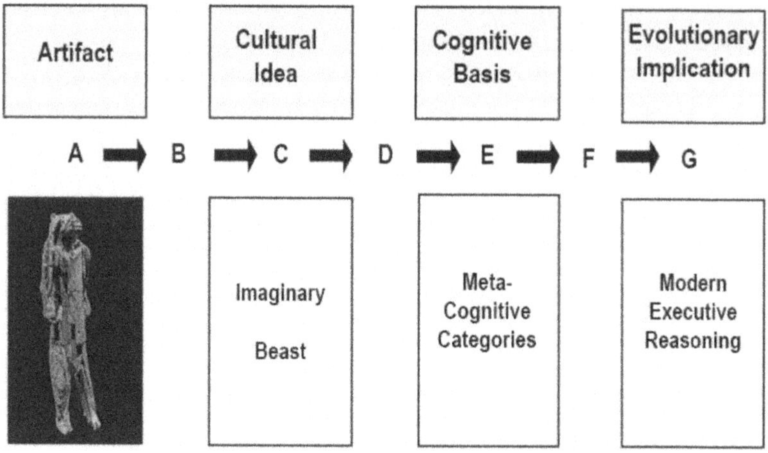

Figure 2 Chart of the therianthrope inference.

to be sound, according to Botha, it must be *pertinent*, *grounded*, and *warranted*. *Pertinence* is the definitional piece; the phenomenon in question must be accurately identified and relevant to the topic under investigation. In this case, a carved figurine of an imaginary animal is just the kind of thing that abstract thinking is expected to traffic in. For the inference to be properly *grounded*, it must be factual and underpinned by an explanatory theory. Modern zoology and paleontology, the scientific knowledge of living and past organisms, ground this inference. Finally, the inference must be *warranted*, which is the logic of science piece to the reasoning. We must explain *how* the data in the left window warrant or justify the conclusion. Warranting requires a testable claim and evidence to support it, which is basic scientific reasoning. "If the artifact has features that do not co-exist in any creature of the natural world, and never have, then the creature represented must be imaginary."

The conclusion of this simple inference becomes the data window on which we base the next inference (CDE) in the chain, and the same requirements of pertinence, grounding, and warranting apply. In this example, the conclusion (E) is that the maker employed a meta-cognitive category to imagine this creature. To be grounded, this inference, too, must be factual and underpinned by an appropriate theory. It is here that cognitive neuroscience enters the reasoning. We know from research in early child development, cognitive psychology, and brain imagery that category formation relies on dedicated neural resources, primarily located in the temporal lobes, that create categories based on resemblances to prototypes (Carey, 2009; Mandler, 2004). Some basic categories are innate—babies are born with them—such as the distinction between animate and inanimate objects. Others are constructed with the aid of experience. In addition to the distinction between animate and inanimate, all humans divide living things into nested taxonomies such that organisms such as lions belong to a separate and distinct category with its own essential (prototypical) qualities (Atran, 1990). The specific taxonomies differ, but the reliance on taxonomic thinking appears to be universal (the natural world itself is characterized by more continuous variation, so the taxonomic bias of humans is a construct not a discovery). With this grounding in cognitive science, we can construct a warranted inference. The imaginary category of lion-man (based on a prototype of lion-man-ness) is not a natural category, but its constituent components are lion head and human body. "If the carver of the lion-man combined separate components from distinct neurally based categories, then he or she would have constructed a higher order category whose prototype extracted and recombined elements of lower order categories." Such thinking about thinking is meta-cognition. The testable hypothesis here is that imaginary categories such as therianthropes require meta-cognition, higher order categories with their own prototypes. Note that here cognitive science provides the grounding in theory and pertinent data, licensing a warranted inference about something required in a prehistoric mind.

The final link in the inference starts with the conclusion about meta-cognitive categories and reaches a further conclusion about the evolutionary status of the mind that conceived the artifact. At this point in the reasoning, the ideational approach would opt for theories of symbolic meaning and the development of religious iconography. ECA turns to theories about the evolution of hominin cognition, especially the higher order cognitive abilities that make up executive reasoning. We ground our inference in the cognitive psychological model of executive functions (Luria, 1973) and working memory (Baddeley, 2007; Baddeley & Hitch, 1974). To shorten our longer argument (Wynn et al., 2009), abstract meta-categories such as lion-man require the resources of modern executive reasoning and working memory capacity. If the carver of Hohlenstein-Stadel used an abstract, meta-category, he or she had a modern mind, or at least that component of modern mindedness.

In a typical presentation of an interpretation, archaeologists rarely lay out all the steps in their inferences. Rhetorically, it is time consuming and potentially tedious (as the reader may have just noticed). It is more common to encounter brief summaries, such as the truncated version we used for our final inference in the preceding paragraph. But in principle it should be possible to specify all the links in a chain of inference, provide the theoretical grounding, and present a warranted inference. If this is not possible, then there is a problem in the reasoning, and the interpretation devolves to mere speculation, the fate of far too many, poorly reasoned claims.

5 Methods of Evolutionary Cognitive Archaeology

Methods are the means by which scholars achieve their goals. Methods select from the varieties of possible evidence and provide frameworks for marshalling that evidence. In Botha's terms, methods are the means for constructing a grounded and warranted inference. "Method" and "methodology" are not synonyms, though some active scholars use them indiscriminately. A methodology is typically a general discussion of how a method or methods yield relevant results, whereas a method is a specific procedure or set of procedures; one is the "how," the other the "what." Some scientific disciplines are very strict about this distinction, but archaeology is not, and it is common in print to see archaeologists describing their "methodology," when they could more simply have used "method." As an example, let us suppose that an archaeologist has the goal of establishing a chronology or dating a site. For the recent past, he or she might choose the method of radiocarbon dating. This now well-established method identifies the variety of evidence (organic material) and the way it marshals evidence (stratigraphically sequenced samples, multiple samples, standard deviations, calibration, etc.). Here, radiocarbon dating is a method. A methodology would discuss the strengths and pitfalls of radiocarbon dating in general. Methods are not techniques, which are instead the practical tools and procedures followed in the lab or the field (in our radiocarbon example this would include extraction of the sample, cleaning, etc.). One can follow a recipe for executing a technique without understanding how the method works. Many an undergraduate's first laboratory experience is doing just this.

Cognitive archaeology relies on a variety of methods. The most productive have been: description/redescription, experimental archaeology, *chaîne opératoire*, and neuroarchaeology.

Description/Redescription

Perhaps, the most common methods of cognitive archaeology are description and redescription. Using concepts and categories grounded in appropriate cognitive theory, the archaeologist identifies attributes that are potentially present in archaeological data and compiles lists of such attributes. He or she can then analyze archaeological assemblages using the attribute list as a kind of key.

DOI: 10.4324/9781003014485-6

The analyses can be qualitative or quantitative. Qualitative attributes can be observed but not measured or counted. Quantitative attributes are numerical and are in the form of measurements or counts. Quantitative attributes often require statistical manipulation to reveal significant patterning (e.g., the average size of artifact A is significantly different from the average size of B), and such statistical manipulation provides a façade of scientism that many archaeologists find comforting. But there is nothing inherently more logical about quantitative attributes than qualitative attributes. If defined properly, both are grounded and repeatable. Of course, the key to persuasive description and redescription lies in the grounding of attributes in cognitive theory. An example from the early days of cognitive archaeology will clarify what we mean.

Piaget and Stone Tools

In the 1970s, Wynn used Jean Piaget's theory of genetic epistemology to ground an interpretation of the evolution of hominin intelligence using stone tools. At the time, Piaget's theory of cognitive development (Piaget, 1960, 1970) dominated developmental psychology, and its description of a sequence of developmental stages made it amenable to studies of evolutionary development. Moreover, Piaget's research had included extensive investigation into children's understanding of spatial relationships, providing an avenue for the analysis of stone tools (Piaget & Inhelder, 1967). The essential task for Wynn was to describe early stone tools using attributes derived from Piaget's analysis of spatial cognition. Previous classifications of early stone tool had been based on presumed function (scraper, chopper), the position of modifications to the artifact (side chopper, end chopper), and sometimes the plan shape (ovate handaxe, triangular cross-section). None of these types or attributes were cognitive in intent, or even tied to explicit spatial relations. Piaget's analysis of children's spatial thinking focused on three general types of spatial relationship—topological, projective, and Euclidean—and identified specific spatial relationships within each that characterized children's actions in space at various points in development. The simplest relationships were topological, including such basic relationships as proximity ("nearbyness") and order. Wynn used these relationships to define attributes, which he then applied to early stone tools from Olduvai Gorge, Tanzania (he performed these analyses in museums in Dar es Salaam and Nairobi). For the relationship of order, in which elements are placed along a contiguous series, Wynn used the attribute of a sequence of unifacial flake removals on the edge of a core or flake. Artifacts with this feature occur in Oldowan assemblages from Bed I in Olduvai Gorge. In a similar fashion, Wynn identified other topological attributes and also projective and Euclidean attributes and deployed them in the description of stone tools from Olduvai, West Natron, and Isimila, all Lower Palaeolithic localities in Tanzania. He was able to describe an evolutionary sequence of increasingly more sophisticated spatial understanding from 1.8 Ma to 300,000 years ago (Wynn, 1979, 1989).

Actualistic Studies and Experimental Archaeology

Artifacts are static objects. Archaeologists cannot directly observe how hominins made, used, and discarded or lost them. All of this must be inferred. There are several methods for warranting these inferences, including technical analyses, residue and microwear analyses, and ethnographic analogy, but often these provide a limited range of information—good for framing hypotheses about the dynamic aspects of artifacts, but rarely persuasive on their own. How can one test such hypotheses? One tried and true test is to examine more sites and artifacts to see if the hypothesis still accounts for the evidence. Another way is through actualistic studies that set out to replicate the use-life of an artifact, or in ambitious cases, replicate the way of life of the hominin responsible. Actualistic studies are also known as experimental archaeology because the intent is to test hypotheses about past procedures, much as chemists test hypotheses about the interaction of elements and molecules using experimental protocols.

In evolutionary cognitive archaeology, actualistic studies encounter a serious limitation that does not apply to other varieties of archaeology. The individuals who replicate prehistoric activities are themselves all modern adults (mostly university students), not premodern hominins. This does not necessarily obviate the conclusions of the analysis, but it does require that the researcher design a project in a way that minimizes the effect of the bias. For example, the researcher could use naïve participants who lack knowledge of the prehistoric past and thus have fewer expectations about how a procedure could work. However, prehistoric actors were not naïve, though many were not modern. Neither were they children, so that avenue is perilous, even if the researcher could pass muster with the institutional review board. Most cognitive archaeologists who use actualistic studies tiptoe through these issues and assume that their modern participants respond in much the way prehistoric hominins did if the results accurately duplicate the archaeological pattern.

Two additional difficulties haunt actualistic studies. The first is the problem of equifinality. Often, several very different procedures or activities will produce the same archaeological pattern. As an example, a hearth from a fire started by capturing natural flame from a brush fire and a hearth from a fire started by friction are indistinguishable archaeologically, yet the cognitive implications of the starting procedures are quite different. Cognitive archaeologists solve this difficulty by settling on the simplest procedure that replicates the pattern, which risks undervaluing ability. However, unless there is other contextual evidence suggesting more sophisticated understandings, it is the only logical way to reason. The second difficulty is the "finished artifact fallacy" (Davidson & Noble, 1989, 1993). Archaeologists often assume that the artifact they have found was the goal of a prehistoric person; that is, someone in the past set out to produce that object. But it turns out that tools often have more complex histories, especially stone tools. A stone knapper may have made a tool for one task, then modified it for another, then lost it, found it again, modified it again, and finally discarded it. Which was the goal? Which the actual tool?

Archaeologists just see the final version. This problem is exacerbated in examples of tools found and repurposed thousands of years later. Whose "thoughts" do we see? Some archaeologists believe this problem is so serious that it cripples cognitive archaeology altogether (McPherron, 2000). It is not necessary to be quite so skeptical, but when formulating actualistic studies, it is important to be aware of this use-life problem and structure the research appropriately.

There are two approaches to actualistic study. The first is largely "ethnographic" in relying heavily on knowledge of preindustrial people in the modern world, especially those living geographically near to the archaeological sample of interest. The second is more experimental in a psychological sense and more narrowly targeted at specific cognitive abilities.

The ethnographic approach, as the term implies, relies heavily on knowledge of living or recent preindustrial people who use or used artifacts similar to those found by archaeologists. The first step is to learn as much as possible about the archaeological artifact's function using an array of well-established techniques such as residue analysis or microwear analysis. The next step is to identify an appropriate ethnographic analogy. The best candidates are people who are living or have lived in the same local environment, with access to the same materials. In ideal cases, the archaeologist observes and interviews people as they make and use the target technology. Very few people in the world today live a truly Palaeolithic lifestyle, especially in regard to technology, so such ideal examples are rare. Reference to ethnographic literature is essential. With this in hand, the archaeologist attempts to replicate the technology using the same materials identified from the ethnographic analog and the archaeological sample. It is almost always necessary to try multiple possibilities before identifying and describing the most likely procedure. Only then can the cognitive archaeologist place the results in the context of cognitive theory and use the replicated activity to warrant conclusions about cognition. Lyn Wadley's classic analysis of Middle Stone Age adhesives is an excellent example (Wadley et al., 2009).

Middle Stone Age Adhesives

The Middle Stone Age (MSA) site of Sibudu Cave in South Africa has yielded remains of stone tools known as segments, which Wadley has demonstrated were components of a projectile technology, probably bow and arrow. While this is itself an interesting cognitive argument, the Wadley et al. (2009) article focused on the adhesives used to haft the segments to the projectile shafts. The adhesive itself has not preserved, except as trace residue on the lithic artifacts. Wadley's discussion is amenable to presentation in Botha's format.

The initial inference—that the segments were components of arrows hafted with adhesives—is warranted through ethnographic knowledge of South African hunters and gatherers and archaeological finds of complete arrows in recent prehistoric sites. Microfractures in the segments themselves corroborate use as projectile components (Wadley et al., 2009). The second inference—the

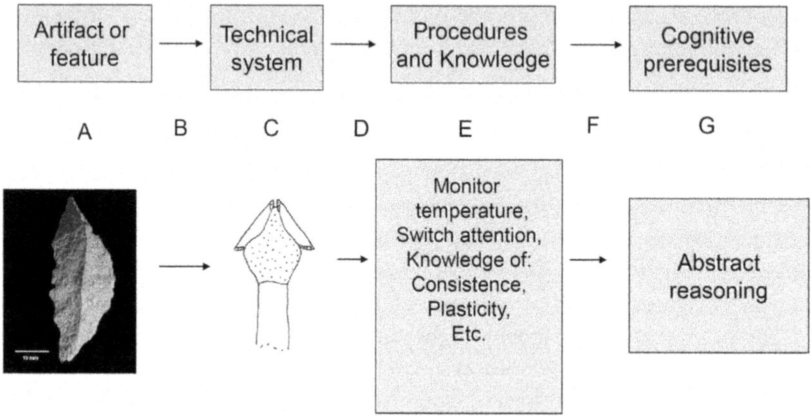

Figure 3 Chart of Wadley's "adhesive inference" (after Wynn, 2009).

knowledge required to produce the adhesive—is warranted through actualistic replication. Residue analysis of the segments themselves revealed microscopic amounts of plant gum and ochre, a mineral pigment. The best gum available in the local environment comes from acacia trees. Wadley et al. tested various combinations and discovered that a malleable adhesive also required the addition of beeswax. They discovered, too, that warming near a fire was essential for dehydrating the adhesive; simple drying did not work. From these replications, Wadley et al. could identify how the Middle Stone Age artisans had to have thought in order to make the adhesive. This included knowledge of necessary qualities of raw material (e.g., plasticity), as well as ability to monitor temperature, and switch attention back and forth between subtasks of the procedure. It is important to note here that these inferences are sound regardless of the species of hominin agent, which presumably was *Homo sapiens*. For the final inference, Wadley et al. turned to an explicit theory of cognitive development, that of Philip Barnard (2010). Barnard's theory is a stage model of cognitive development based on information processing. The final stage of cognitive development includes the ability to process two levels of meaning simultaneously. Wadley et al. suggest that the task switching necessary to produce the adhesive required this kind of abstract mindedness, and thus, the Sibudu adhesive makers had fully modern minds. The inference about task switching was warranted by the actualistic replication of the adhesive (Wynn, 2009).

A second variety of actualistic replication draws on the techniques of controlled experimentation used in psychology. The first step is to isolate an ability of interest and develop a hypothesis amenable to controlled experimentation. The researcher then devises an experimental protocol or protocols that test predictions of the hypothesis, including explicit standards for evaluating results. He or she then recruits participants, who follow the prescribed protocols in controlled environments. Video documentation is now common both as a way to store raw data and as a permanent record available to other researchers. The researcher then evaluates results using the initial explicit measures and applies statistical techniques to evaluate significance. As with all deductive reasoning, experimentation can reject a hypothesis but never logically prove a hypothesis. Positive results merely support the hypothesis.

Stone Knapping and Social Learning

Morgan et al. (2015) published the results of an experimental comparison of various styles of learning applied to stone knapping. They were primarily interested in the role of teaching in social learning. Several archaeologists (including Coolidge & Wynn!) had suggested that early hominins had learned stone knapping through observation of skilled adults, but not linguistic instruction. Others disagreed, arguing instead that active teaching of some kind was required. Morgan et al. first narrowed the question to a specific hypothesis: "Oldowan stone tool production could have generated selection for complex forms of social transmission that enhanced the fidelity of information transmission" (Morgan et al., 2015, p. 2). They then designed a series of protocols to evaluate five different varieties of learning: (1) reverse engineering (researchers supplied participants with stone hammers, cores, and flakes but no other information); (2) imitation/emulation (participants observed a skilled knapper produce flakes); (3) basic teaching (teachers positioned materials and participants' hands); (4) gestural teaching (teacher gestured and pointed to direct attention); and (5) verbal instruction. As one means of judging efficacy, the experiment arranged participants into "chains"—after learning the basic knapping gesture a participant became the skilled expert for the next "generation" of participants. If social learning had been effective, the next generation should also learn efficiently and be able in their turn to pass it on again. The protocol also measured skill through evaluation of knapping products, including number and size of flakes and number of successful blows. "Across numerous measures of individual performance, we consistently found that teaching and language, but not imitation or emulation, enhanced the acquisition of stone knapping skills relative to reverse engineering" (p. 3). Moreover, only teaching (gestural and verbal) provided sufficient understanding for effective knapping to pass down more than one link down the chain of generations. The authors then use the results to discuss implications for early stone knapping and the establishment of cultural traditions.

Ethnographic and experimental approaches to actualistic study have rather different but equally important roles to play in cognitive archaeology. Ethnographic approaches such as Wadley's expand the data available for interpretation and test assumptions about prehistoric technology. The cognitive interpretations resemble those of cognitive anthropology—rich in detail and thus less amenable to quantitative analysis. Experimental approaches such as Morgan et al. have greater validity and reliability but are narrowly focused and lack the rich detail of the ethnographic approach. Both provide insights into past cognition and, as we will show, are often the initial steps in other methods.

Chaînes Opératoires

Chaînes opératoires (operational or procedural chains) are descriptions of sequences of actions, typically related to tool use and technical activities. French social anthropologist Leroi-Gourhan coined the term 70 or so years ago, and the documentation of *chaînes operatoires* became a component of an anthropology of technology that focused on the social context of action. It also became an important organizational concept for French Palaeolithic archaeology (Andouze & Karlin, 2017). Initially, and still in some quarters, the use of *chaînes opératoires* included a commitment to its theoretical stance regarding the role of social context in technology, and indeed, one of the more sophisticated analyses of Levallois lithic reduction (Schlanger, 1996) took this approach. But for good or ill archaeologists are a practical lot, and it is now more common to encounter *chaînes opératoires* shorn of their initial theoretical coat and reconfigured with a different theoretical stance (or in some cases none at all, at least explicitly).

The goal of a *chaîne opératoire* is a comprehensive step-by-step account of the use-life of an artifact or feature from conception to discard. Artifacts and features, however, are frozen at the point in time they were lost, discarded, or abandoned. Archaeologists must infer any sequential information they might carry, and there are several methods that archaeologists use to warrant these inferences. The first is simple common sense: discard follows use, which follows manufacture, and so on. If one adds knowledge of the context of use gleaned from the archaeological record, common sense can provide more elaborate sequences including steps involving transport distances and curation. However, common sense is limited and potentially deceptive; it is after all based in the analyst's preconceptions about the nature of human activities, a notoriously weak warrant. Most serious applications of *chaînes opératoires* warrant their inferences using technical analyses or actualistic studies. For example, close visual analysis of ceramic remains can reveal manufacturing procedures, including step-by-step accounts of mixing the clay and temper, techniques for starting a vessel, adding material, decorating, firing, and so on. With more sophisticated microscopic and chemical analyses, one can often identify sources for the clay. The result is a far more reliable account of the *chaîne opératoire*, one that can warrant inferences about the potter's decision-making. For Palaeolithic studies, one of the more persuasive forms of technical analysis is refitting. In stone knapping, every successful strike produces a flake that is unique in size and shape and also often in the color and pattern of the raw material. With time and patience, an analyst can, in principle, refit all the flakes from a core back together into the original clast, a kind of three-dimensional jigsaw puzzle. It is then possible to reverse the procedure and describe the exact sequence of flake removals—and decisions—followed by the original knapper.

Much depends on how much of a lithic episode remains at one location to be found and documented later by an archaeologist. In ideal cases, such as the 2.3 Ma site Lokalalei 2C, almost all the flakes were present, which enabled the analysts to completely refit multiple cores (Delagnes & Roche, 2005). However, even in cases where only a few flakes fit together, the analysis is almost always worth the effort.

Actualistic studies often warrant inferences about *chaînes opératoires*. In a tour-de-force of archaeological analysis, Naama Goren-Inbar et al. started with the charred remains of water-lily seeds excavated from 800,000-year-old deposits at Gesher Benot Ya'aqov. Using ethnographic accounts from India, and experimental replication using modern plants, they were able to reconstruct the outlines of the *chaîne opératoire* used in gathering and processing the resource. One of the indispensable steps was drying, a step that required several days. This interruption in the temporal continuity of the procedure has important cognitive implications (Alperson-Afil et al., 2020).

There is no standard format for presenting *chaînes opératoires*, which makes comparison difficult, even impossible. Most interpretations involving *chaînes opératoires* are thus wholly self-contained. This makes evolutionary analyses problematic. A major exception to this caveat is the work of Miriam Haidle.

Cognigrams

In a series of articles and book chapters, Haidle and her collaborators have applied a consistent *chaîne opératoire* technique to a variety of examples, and the result has been a persuasive description of the evolution of technical cognition (Haidle, 2009; Lombard & Haidle, 2012; Lombard et al., 2018). Haidle based her technique in comparative studies, initially contrasting chimpanzee technical problem-solving with that of early hominins. She drew her theoretical grounding from the classic studies of chimpanzees made by Wolfgang Köhler. From Köhler's work, she identified an analytical concept that could apply to any technical activity—problem-solution distance, which is the number and nature of links between an initial perception of need and fulfillment of the goal. From this basic orienting stance, she derived a set of concepts to be used for parsing activity streams into cognitively relevant behavioral units centered on the perspective of the tool using agent. There are five steps to Haidle's analysis: identify foci of attention, identify perception of needs, identify the smallest action units (steps), identify effects of one focus on another, and parse the action stream into phases of "tightly linked actions" (Haidle, 2010; Lombard & Haidle, 2012). The output of this analysis is a "cognigram" that graphically presents the foci, steps, and phases of the activity. These cognigrams provide a quick, visual means of comparing technical activities to one another, but they also incorporate the detailed reasoning of the five analytical steps and thus reward detailed examination. Here, we present two examples:

Haidle's cognigrams make one point abundantly clear: describing technical activities is difficult and laborious. Even with a well-stipulated five-step

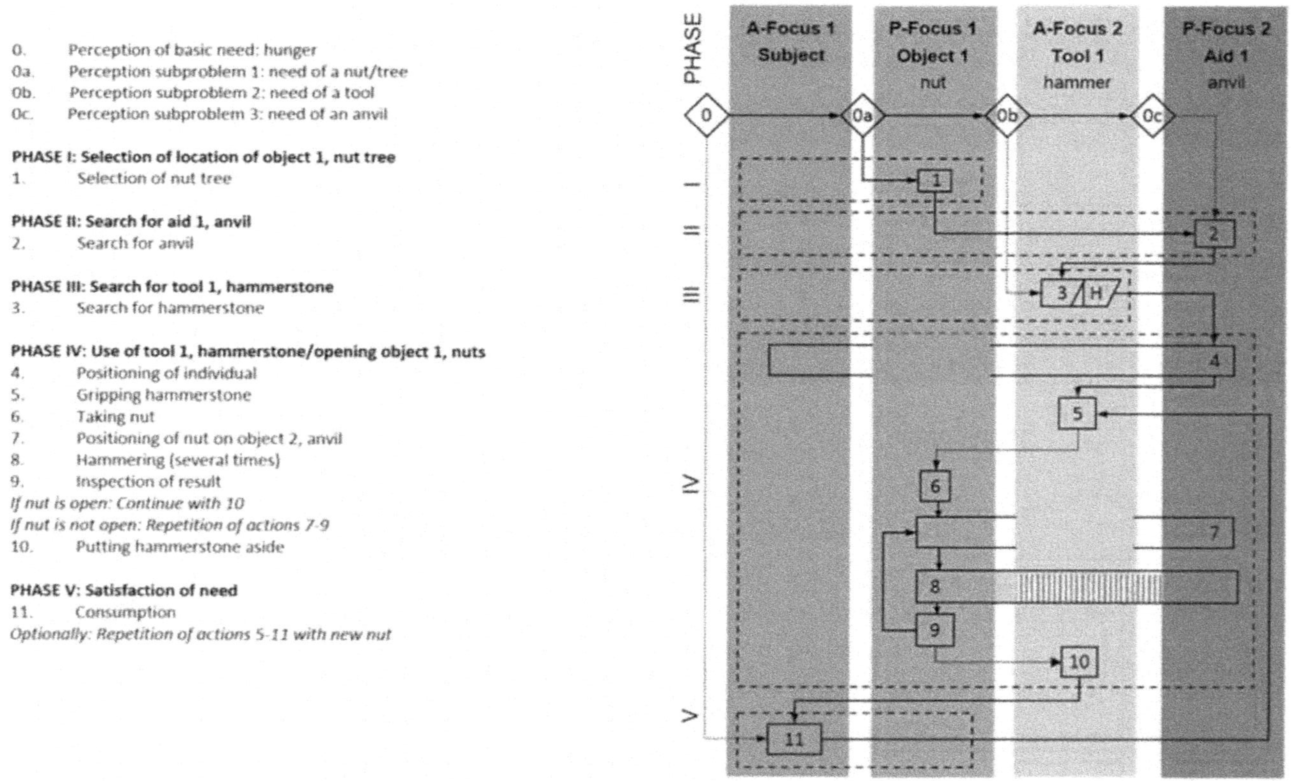

Figure 4 Cognigram of chimpanzee nut cracking. After Lombard et al., 2019.

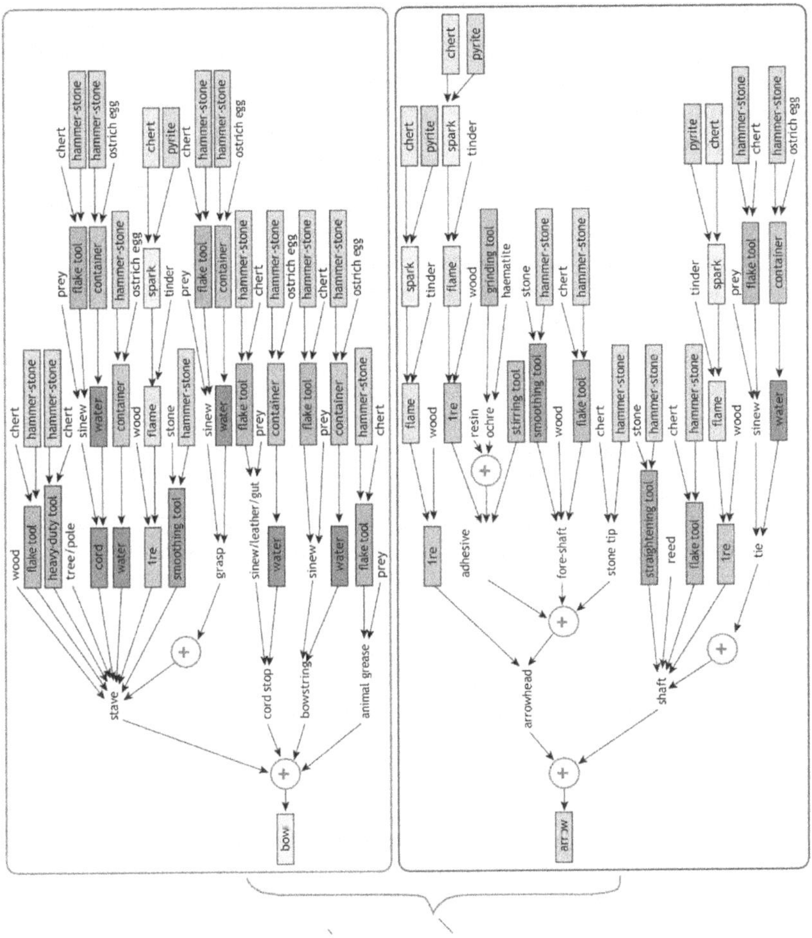

Figure 5 Chart summarizing the multiple cognigrams necessary to describe the production of a bow and arrow. After Lombard & Haidle, 2012.

analytical procedure and well-defined graphic units, compiling a cognigram requires a number of comparatively arbitrary decisions. Identifying foci and steps is a real challenge, even for an activity as comparatively simple as chimpanzee nut cracking. The technique is also minimally grounded in a theoretical sense. Köhler's work was historically significant, but it no longer underpins active research in comparative psychology. Problem-solution distance is more promising but alone functions more as a descriptive guide than a true cognitive interpretation. However, Haidle's cognigrams are far-and-away the most useful cognitively based *chaînes opératoires* available. Their clarity and comprehensiveness are amenable to alternative theoretical grounding, resulting in warranted inferences unspecified by Haidle herself. For example, attention switching is a component of cognitive control in Baddeley's working memory model, and because cognigrams incorporate shifts in attention, they potentially document developments in cognitive control.

Neuroarchaeology

The most ambitious and potentially impactful method in cognitive archaeology is neuroarchaeology—the documentation of neural activation patterns that underpin archaeologically identified activities (Stout et al., 2000). The method incorporates actualistic studies and brain imaging technologies of various kinds. The goal is twofold. First, the method strives to describe neural activation patterns for activities of interest. Neuroscience itself has shown only modest interest in the activities that archaeologists study, and one cannot go to the brain science literature and find descriptions of brain activity underpinning pottery making or spear manufacture. Neuroarchaeology thus expands the scope of neuroscience in important ways. Second, by describing neural activation patterns produced by proxies making artifacts typical of different points in hominin evolution, one can begin to document the evolution of these neural activation patterns. This obviously has great relevance to cognitive archaeology.

The method is the most complex, time consuming, and expensive in the cognitive archaeologist's toolbox. It begins with actualistic replication of an activity of interest, either ethnographic/experiential or experimental. Given the experimental paradigms required for the neural imaging component, most studies are fairly narrowly experimental. Often, this actualistic step involves extensive training of participants as a means of standardizing response. Although studies of individual participants have been influential (Stout et al., 2015), reliability requires larger samples. And, of course, all the caveats adhering to actualistic studies apply here as well. The second step in neuroarchaeology is neural imaging. Typically, a participant performs a set of standard actions for a set number of repetitions or time periods and then moves immediately to a scanner of some kind that records brain activation. Given the sensitivity of most kinds of scans, the participants must remain still for the scan itself. Thus, there is a delay between the action and the scan; however, this delay is not as limiting as it seems because neural activation patterns, or at least the indirect effect measured by the scanners, fade over the course of minutes, not seconds. An alternative approach is to have participants visualize action when they are in the scanner. With scan results in hand, the analyst compares activation patterns to a baseline state to identify regions made active by the experimental task and/or compares the result to patterns produced by other activities. With multiple participants, the analyst can compile an average activation pattern and increase the reliability of the result.

Brain imaging technologies do not record neuron firings per se. Instead, they measure correlated effects of neural activity. Electroencephalography (EEG), for example, detects the electrical signals and oscillations in the electrical signal produced by neural activity. Positron emission tomography (PET) and functional magnetic resonance imaging (fMRI) detect changes in blood flow to the brain. Increases in neural activation produce increases in blood flow, and the regions of the brain that activate during a task will have increased blood flow. PET detects this change in blood flow by means of a radioactive tracer injected into the blood stream of a participant. Although a now classic study of stone knapping used this technique (Stout et al., 2000), its invasive nature limits its usefulness. The fMRI scanner detects the BOLD signature—blood oxygenation-level dependent—which measures changes in the ratio of oxygenated to deoxygenated blood via changes in magnetic signature. These techniques do not detect individual neuron firings but instead measure the response of regions of varying size. The resolution of EEG is determined by the number of electrodes placed on the scalp (anywhere from 4 to 256, with 30 being typical). Thus, the spatial resolution of EEG is very coarse. However, EEG has the great advantage of measuring and recording changes in electrical activity in real time. fMRI has much greater resolution in location, typically presenting activation states of "voxels," each of which has a brain tissue volume of 3 ×3 ×3 mm. Each voxel contains thousands of neurons. fMRI results are presented graphically with different colors for different activation states. The resulting "picture" of brain activity is often quite attractive.

Brains and Handaxes

The research program of Dietrich Stout et al. is perhaps the best current example of neuroarchaeological research (Stout & Chaminade, 2007, 2012; Stout et al., 2000, 2009, 2015; Stout & Hecht, 2017; Hecht et al., 2014). The focus is on hominin cognitive evolution in general using actualistic stone tool manufacture and fMRI. A 2015 study focused on the possible role of cognitive control and semantic knowledge in the production of Acheulean handaxes (Stout et al., 2015). For the actualistic component, expert stone knappers trained six novice participants how to knap basic Oldowan-like flakes, Acheulean style handaxes, and Levallois cores. Training and practice occurred over a 22-month period. The imaging component employed standard fMRI and also fcMRI, which traces water diffusion along white matter tracks and thus measures connectivity between regions. Because participants must remain still during scans, they could not knap as the scan took place (napping is another matter). Instead, Stout et al. asked the participants to evaluate videos of rotating flakes and cores on which possible points of impact were indicated by colored dots and a predicted result by white area. The participants judged whether the proposed blow would produce the suggested outcome, and also whether the indicated spot was the best choice. Such judgments reflected the participants understanding of the knapping process.

Fig. 6 reproduces a figure from the original publication. In this figure, Stout et al. summarize the interaction of time and technology in the experimental

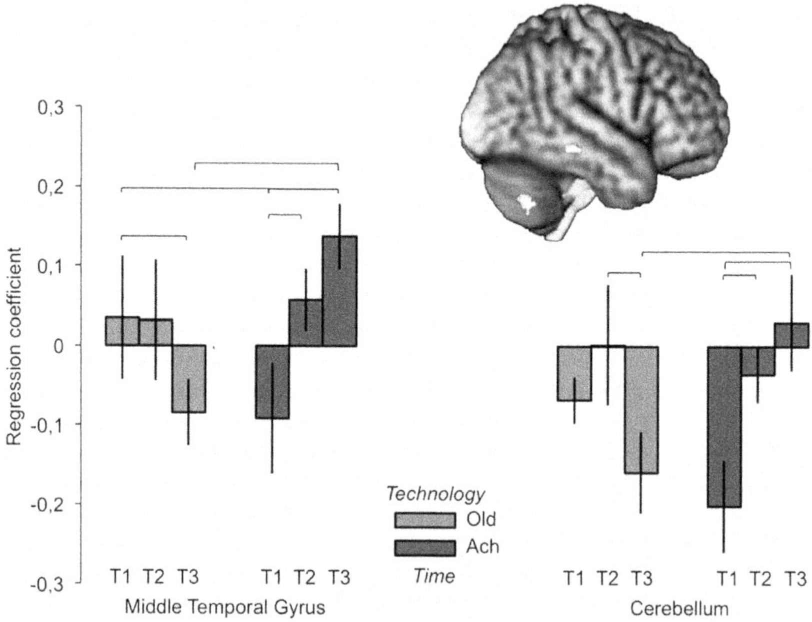

Figure 6 Chart comparing brain activation in production of Oldowan and Acheulean stone tools. After Stout et al., 2015.

results. Here, time measures three different points (and scans) in learning to knap (beginning, middle, and end). Technology contrasts handaxe manufacture (prediction and strategy) in dark gray with assessing simple Oldowan flake manufacture in light gray. The brain image identifies two areas of neural activation: the middle temporal gyrus (MTG) and the cerebellum. The graphs summarize the intensity of the effect. What is clear from the graph is that the activation of the MTG increases with training (from T1 to T3). The authors interpret this result as reflecting the increased importance of semantic knowledge concerning how to make a handaxe. No significant effect accompanied assessment of the Oldowan flakes and cores.

Section II

Core Issues in Evolutionary Cognitive Archaeology

6 Memory

What is the relationship between learning and memory? Learning is a knowledge or skill that is acquired by instruction, practice, experience, or study. Cognitive psychologist Endel Tulving (1995) noted that memory always presupposes some learning process, and the word *memory* implies the retention of that information. Discussions of learning and memory usually begin with the forms of learning and the forms of memory.

Forms of Learning

There are said to be two forms of learning: nonassociative and associative (e.g., Kandel, 2009). Nonassociative learning is the older of the two (Bronfman et al., 2016), dating back to the first forms of life, the single-cell prokaryotes, about 3.9 billion years ago. There are two forms of nonassociative learning: habituation and sensitization (e.g., d'Isa et al., 2011). In habituation, the strength or probability of a response is *reduced* by repeated presentation of a stimulus. This is the simplest form of learning, and it has been observed in nearly all animals and some plants (e.g., Abramson & Chicas-Mosier, 2016). In sensitization, the strength or probability of a response is *increased* by a repeated stimulus; thus, sensitization means that an organism becomes increasingly more sensitive or more responsive to a particular stimulus. It is also important to note that the term "nonassociative" is a misnomer, as there is an obvious association or relationship between the stimulus and response. However, the name might imply that the two nonassociative forms of learning, habituation and sensitization, are *not* the two forms of associative learning, classical and operant conditioning.

Associative learning has two major forms: classical conditioning and operant conditioning. Classical conditioning, which is also known as Pavlovian conditioning, is attributed to the Russian physiologist and Nobel laureate Ivan Pavlov (1849–1936), who trained a dog to salivate (the conditioned response or CR) to a sound like a bell (the conditioned stimulus or CS) by pairing the bell with food (the unconditioned stimulus or UCS). In the classical conditioning paradigm, "natural" or "reflexive pairings" like the sight and smell of food (UCS) to a dog elicits the unconditioned response (UCR), that is saliva. It is important to note that the dog does not

DOI: 10.4324/9781003014485-8

have to learn this association, as it is considered a reflex, although the pairing had to have been initially learned and retained over evolutionary time.

The second form of associative learning is operant conditioning where a behavior of the organism either increases or decreases in frequency based on its subsequent pairing with a stimulus. A reinforcing stimulus increases the probability of a response in the future. Punishment decreases the probability of a response.

Forms of Memory

There are many more classification systems for memory than there are for learning (Kandel, 2009; Squire, 2004). One such system is based on recall time after learning and consists of sensory memory, short-term memory, and long-term memory. Sensory memory is not really a type of memory recall per se but consists of sensory perceptions (usually visual or auditory) that persist very briefly—seconds or less. Short-term memory is defined as the recall of recently learned information over somewhat longer periods, typically seconds or minutes. Long-term memory is the recall of information over hours, days, years, or one's lifetime. While the time parameter may appear to be arbitrary, the neurological changes over time are different between the three forms. The initial encoding is not different (at least for verbal materials).

Cognitive psychologists divide long-term memory into two categories: explicit memory and implicit memory. Explicit memory is the recall for facts, words, meanings, and events. It is also called declarative memory or semantic memory, and those two terms are completely synonymous, for humans at least. Implicit memory is the recall for skills or procedures, like riding a bicycle, juggling, or stone knapping. The latter are also called procedural memories. One unique type of explicit memory, which is known to be phenomenologically different than a declarative memory, is episodic memory, which consists of the recall of whole scenes with *what*, *where*, and *when* characteristics (e.g., Tulving, 1995). Episodic memory has even been attributed to animals like scrub jays and foxes (e.g., Allen & Fortin, 2013). It is important to note that the episode must also carry sufficient emotional valence (or sufficient meaning) to a human or other animal. The emotional valence of a memory and the ability to recall it are inextricably intertwined because the formation of the coding of an episodic memory depends on how emotionally arousing the memory is or how emotionally meaningful it is.

A subtype of episodic memory is an autobiographical memory (Rubin, 1999), which is an episodic memory with a strong sense of self in its recall, and thus, autobiographical memories may be restricted to humans. One subtype of autobiographical memory is a flashbulb memory (e.g., Winograd & Neisser, 2006). Although the term is now archaic, it referred to a time when cameras could only take pictures in low light situations if there was a sudden but intense flash of light from a bulb. Flashbulb memories are typically restricted to highly emotional events, like natural disasters, war scenes, terrorist acts (like 9/11 for

Americans), and other types of catastrophes. In the recall of such memories, the person can usually recall the place, time, date, and where they were while witnessing the event. These memories are also referred to as one-trial learning, as it only takes one very traumatic experience to persist for a lifetime.

Working Memory

There are at least two popular understandings of working memory. One is a generic version that can be defined as the ability to hold information in one's attention and make decisions while inhibiting irrelevant internal and external stimuli. The other version is a multicomponent learning and memory model proposed by British psychologist Alan Baddeley (Baddeley & Hitch, 1974; Baddeley, 2001, 2012) that incorporates both implicit and explicit memory. First, he hypothesized the metaphorical existence of a *central executive* that attended to relevant stimuli consonant with short- and long-term goals, processed information, made decisions, and inhibited interference. A similar metaphorical structure to the central executive had been earlier proposed by Russian neuropsychologist Alexander Luria (1966), who hypothesized that the frontal lobes were largely responsible for "executive functions," which included the ability to plan and organize tasks, sequence tasks, and action inhibition (e.g., delayed gratification). Baddeley also hypothesized that working memory had two memory subsystems and a multimodal memory component. The *phonological loop* subsystem consisted of a phonological store, which briefly holds sounds (about 2 seconds) in order to determine their meaning, and the vocal (subvocal) articulatory processor, which acts like a rehearsal mechanism, where sounds or words are repeated in one's mind or vocally to store them in long-term memory. The second subsystem, the *visuospatial sketchpad*, temporarily holds visual and spatial information, and it can recall and even simulate story-like memories (also known as episodic memory). In addition to the two subsystems, Baddeley proposed a memory component serving at the behest of the central executive. He labeled it the *episodic buffer*, a kind of short-term memory that integrated multimodal sensory information from the phonological loop and the visuospatial sketchpad.

On the Nature of Forgetting

Schacter (2012) and his colleagues (e.g., Schacter & Addis, 2007; Schacter et al., 2011) do *not* view forgetting and the imperfections of memory recall as evidence of a defective or flawed system. They did see them as evidence of a "dynamic memory system that flexibly incorporates relevant new information" (Schacter, 2012, p. 2). He and his colleagues proposed that the original function of episodic memory was not for the perfect recall of an episode. Rather, they hypothesized that evolutionary value of an episodic memory was that pertinent details of an episode could be recalled, reconstructed, and reassembled and then used to simulate alternative future scenarios and outcomes in those various scenarios. Just as Shepard (1997) had proposed earlier, these thought experiments were much safer than actual trial and sometimes fatal error.

It may also be likely that greater working memory capacity would allow for more reflections and comparisons of past experiences, which would enhance the probability of mental models that were more likely to be successful than other in solving novel problems and anticipating future events. Individuals could then actively choose a future action or create alternative actions, rather than simply choosing the highest path of probable success. Individuals could still benefit from choosing alternatives based solely on past successes and failures, but an individual who could actively compare multiple simulated scenarios and combine them into novel actions would be at an advantage. The ability to solve novel problems with novel solutions is the definition of fluid intelligence, and empirical studies have demonstrated the strong association between working memory capacity and fluid intelligence.

We will revisit this concept of an enhancement in working memory as one of the clearest of cognitive differences between Phase 2 and Phase 3 of hominin cognitive evolution. We will also present the innovative technologies of bows and arrows and snares and traps as part of the archaeological evidence for enhanced working memory in Phase 3 of Chapter 14.

7 Technical Cognition

Over the last two centuries, archaeologists have acquired a vast data set of past technologies: millions of stone tools and broken pots, thousands of ovens and hearths, houses and shelters, and countless curios of unknown use or meaning. And through experimentation and replication, we have a good understanding of the ways in which many of these technologies worked. But psychology's understanding of the cognition governing tool use is not equally robust. There are several reasons for this dearth, but two are especially relevant to cognitive archaeology. The first is the low esteem that academics have for tool use. Most academics, including cognitive scientists, consider rhetoric and mathematical reasoning to be the pinnacles of human thought and the everyday basis for scientific investigation. They consider plumbing and auto maintenance to be necessary real-world distractions but not as worthy of serious investigation. Thus, Western science knows far more about how children learn math than how they learn to bake bread. The second reason is more insidious. Most people educated in Western schools have a "folk theory" of technical cognition that is misleading. It is what one might call the "great inventor" theory, and it goes something like this: people think about tools using mental imagery ("representations" in cognitive science terms) and when confronted with a technical problem they employ a "mental simulation" in which they envision a way wherein their imagined tools will solve the problem. Sometimes these mental simulations yield new solutions and technologies that produce progressive change. However, this is not how people think when they use tools, at least not very often. If we want to study the evolution of technical cognition—and we do—we need to acquire a better model of technical cognition than the folk theory. Our first step is to describe what is entailed when a person uses a tool.

Think for a moment about apprenticeship. In the twenty-first century, it is still the system of learning by which many novices acquire technical knowledge and skill, and its features reveal important clues to technical cognition. An apprenticeship is an extended period (often years) during which a novice learns a set of technical procedures by first observing a master or masters at work, followed by trial-and-error attempts, followed by extensive practice until he or she achieves an acceptable level of performance, as judged by a master. The essential components of apprenticeship are observation and practice.

DOI: 10.4324/9781003014485-9

Verbal instruction is secondary; indeed, in some apprenticeships, it is forbidden altogether. Verbal instruction is secondary because technical knowledge is primarily nonlinguistic, consisting instead of embodied procedures and action sequences generated and remembered through muscular/motor patterns and motor memories. This, by the way, is why accessing fix-it tips on the internet is often so frustrating; the solutions on offer consist of verbal descriptions that cannot provide the motor/procedural knowledge one acquires only through practice. But it is not just bodily practice and motor memory. Tools themselves play an active role in technical thinking and apprenticeship. Tools, especially hand tools, become extensions of the body. Through repetition and practice, tools become components of the neurocognitive system itself, including the neural wiring that underpins all learning. How we understand a task is determined to some degree by the tools we use. Of course, we can and do talk and write about tools and technology and can even learn a few things about tool use this way. But no one has ever learned to be a blacksmith or even fix an automobile by simply reading a book. We can read about knowing, but we cannot know until we try.

This brief account of apprenticeship tells us that our folk theory of technical thinking does not capture the true nature of technical cognition. Although we can think about tools using the "envision a goal; think of a tool; execute" model of our folk theory, this is but one component of technical cognition and arguably not the most important. There is another domain of "thinking" that does not consist of mental images or simulations and is far older in an evolutionary sense.

Archaeologists have only recently come to appreciate the domain features of technical cognition and there are several competing theories that govern formal interpretations of the past. We summarize three.

Material Engagement Theory

Material Engagement Theory (MET) dispenses with the notion of internal thoughts and simulations altogether (Malafouris, 2013). Thinking consists not just of neural activity "in the head" but also of bodies and tools. A blind person's cane is a famous example. A blind individual quite literally perceives the world through the tip of a cane; the tool has become a component of mind. Another example is an abacus. An adept user does not even think "about" the abacus, but through it; it becomes a component of reasoning itself. Malafouris suggests that examples like these are not odd curiosities but instead are quite normal components of our thinking, and if we aspire to understand the evolution of the human mind, we must understand the active role of tools in human thinking. Thus, when MET considers stone tools, it emphasizes how early hominins thought *through* those artifacts, not the nature of human thoughts *about* the artifacts. In a compelling discussion of the earliest beads from Blombos Cave in South Africa, Malafouris described how people might have used the beads to create a more sophisticated form of social agency. The beads were thus a mechanism for social thinking, not just a reflection of social identity. MET applications to the deep past are thus far few, but as we will see, the approach has great potential to decode some puzzles, such as why hominins began making handaxes 1.79 million years ago.

The "Two Network" Model of Neuropsychology

The most explicit neurocognitive models of tool use are derived from neuropsychological research, which documents patterns of neural/behavioral loss caused by injury or pathology. The gold standard of neuropsychology is double dissociation. Let's say patient A has left frontal lobe damage and loses the ability to speak but still understands spoken sentences. This suggests, but does not prove, that language relies on at least two separate brain areas. Patient B has left temporal lobe damage and can no longer understand speech but retains an ability to speak. This double dissociation confirms that speech execution and speech understanding rely on distinct neural resources (recognized first 160 years ago by Paul Broca). Tool use also presents a double dissociation, though the pattern is not as localized. Some individuals with parietal lobe damage lose the ability to manipulate familiar tools in an appropriate way even though they can identify their functions verbally. For example, a patient understands that matches are for creating fire but cannot perform the appropriate action to get one to light. He or she has lost what Goldenberg labels "manipulation knowledge" (Goldenberg, 2012; Goldenberg & Spatt, 2009). Other patients retain the ability to manipulate a tool appropriately but lose an ability to identify its purpose or use it to solve problems. According to Goldenberg, these patients have a deficit in "mechanical reasoning." This distinction makes sense of features of apprenticeship, where physical practice establishes and enhances manipulation knowledge, and project experience builds a framework of mechanical reasoning. Note that this neuropsychological model grants no role to the tools themselves; the focus is on brains as agents governing all aspects of technical behavior. But the fact that the brain deploys two relatively distinct sets of neural resources to support tool use is certainly provocative and must be considered in any account of technical cognition.

Expert Performance

MET focuses on tools as components of technical thinking and minimizes the role of the brain; neuropsychology focuses on neural resources but grants no active role to the tools themselves. Are there approaches that incorporate both? The answer is a qualified yes, largely because the proposed models are in the initial stages of development (recall that academics have tended to disrespect tool use). Dietrich Stout et al. have been using experimental replication and neural imaging to investigate the evolution of technical cognition, and their approach recognizes the plasticity of neural networks and an active role for tools (Stout & Hecht, 2017). Francois Osiurak and Emanuelle Reynaud have recently proposed a model of technical cognition that incorporates both neuropsychological data and an active role for tools (Osiurak et al., 2020; Osiurak & Reynaud, 2020). Here, however, we advocate for an approach we have developed that is based in neurocognitive models for what psychologists label "expert performance."

Imagine a chess master playing several games simultaneously while blindfolded. This is a seemingly impossible feat; after all, if short-term memory is limited to 5–7 items held in attention (Miller, 1956), and if long-term memory requires multiple exposures over time, how could he or she track the movement of 32 pieces on the 64 squares of multiple boards without being able to see them? The answer is that an expert relies on a variety of thinking that uses well-learned knowledge frameworks to enhance attention and working memory. Expert performance has several salient features:

(1) The expert performs tasks quickly with a high level of accuracy, rarely making unforced errors.
(2) The expert performs in-depth assessments of task problems with little apparent effort.
(3) Expertise is largely automatic and once initiated requires little in the way of active attention.
(4) Expert performance is resistant to fading. Relevant information does not lose coherence over time.
(5) An expert can be interrupted and return to a task with little or no loss of relevant information.
(6) An expert can learn new task-relevant information very rapidly.
(7) Expertise is limited to a narrow domain of behavior and does not transfer easily, even to related domains (e.g., chess to Go).
(8) Expertise requires years and thousands of repetitions to acquire.

Chess and board games are not the only domains of expertise. Psychologists have studied expertise in musical performance, medical diagnosis, individual and team sports, and acting. All share the features listed previously. Psychologists have paid less attention to tool use, for reasons mentioned earlier, but our understanding of mastery in craftsmanship matches up nicely. Technical expertise is most like expertise in sport. Both incorporate motor procedures, postures, and execution sequences in their problem-solving and both require years of physical practice.

There are several influential models of expert cognition. All of them focus on what Alessandro Guida (Guida et al., 2012) terms "knowledge structures" [Ericsson (1999) uses "retrieval structure" and Gobet (2016) uses "template"]. A knowledge structure is a well-learned set of related "cues," each of which is tied to a much larger set of information (psychologists use the term "chunk") stored in long-term memory. For example, the cue "King's Indian Defense" instantly accesses the location of 32 pieces on the chess board over the course of several moves. The chess player activates the knowledge structure "chess openings" when beginning a game and need only hold the cue "King's Indian Defense" in working memory to have instant access to large amount of task relevant information. This information need not be verbal. In the sport of fencing, an opponent's posture, distance, and blade position cue well-learned automatic motor responses consisting of parries, counterattacks, or retreats learned laboriously over years of practice. In blacksmithing, the color, sound, and resistance of heated metal as it is hammered cue an appropriate sequence of blows, turns, and reheatings. Because cues and responses are very well-learned, unforced mistakes are rare and response is seemingly instantaneous. And because almost all the information is stored in long-term memory, the expert can be distracted and return to a task with little loss of information. As Guida describes it, "when an individual has acquired expertise in a domain, part of LTM [long-term memory] can be accessed rapidly and reliably and therefore used as WM" (Guida et al., 2012, p. 224). In a sense, expertise takes advantage of the strengths of long-term memory and working memory and circumvents their weaknesses. Long-term memory has a huge capacity but is typically less reliable and takes time and effort to acquire; working memory has a small capacity but can react quickly and reliably. Neuroimaging confirms that experts rely on LTM resources when executing WM memory problems in their domains of expertise. There are downsides to expertise. It is difficult to acquire, and it does not transfer well. An expert pianist is not automatically an expert violinist (or even an expert harpsichordist). Expertise is not inherently creative. Experts demonstrate impressive flexibility in response to changing conditions because they draw on a huge array of well-learned responses. Creativity taps different neural resources (Wynn & Coolidge, 2014).

Thus far, psychological models of expertise have taken an implicitly Cartesian view of the mind in which expert thinking occurs in the head, contra Malafouris's insistence that bodies and tools are active components of thought. But these models are open to the incorporation of embodied and extended resources without doing damage to their interpretive power. Tools act as cues to well-learned perceptual and motor patterns. They also organize motor responses. Indeed, if we take ethnographic accounts of technical cognition into consideration, the knowledge structures of technical expertise consist almost entirely of embodied routines of motor memory, and the active organizational power of tools and materials. As Charles Keller described it (Keller & Keller, 1996), the availability of metal stock and the tools at hand in the shop are part of the thought processes of the blacksmith. They are real components of the blacksmith's knowledge structures, not just metaphors. There are, of course, neural correlates to expertise, especially in the temporal lobes and the cerebellum, but they do not generate "thoughts" in the sense of internal images and representations. When expanded by incorporation of embodied and extended resources, the cognitive model of expert cognition provides a powerful model for investigating technical cognition and its evolution.

The expert cognition model enables archaeologists to describe technical cognition with terms and concepts that have greater cognitive validity than commonsense terms such as complexity and sophistication. Instead of simply asserting that technology X is more complex than Y, one can compare the respective knowledge structures, including their inherent organization and the roles played by tools themselves. In Botha's terms, expert cognition provides the grounding. The methods of cognitive archaeology provide the warrants. *Chaînes opératoires*, Haidle's cognigrams in particular, are perhaps the most comprehensive approach (Wynn et al., 2017), but actualistic archaeology and neuroarchaeology are also appropriate methods. The result is a description of technical cognition amenable to comparing hominins to one another and to nonhuman primates.

Neandertal Expertise

The richness of the Neandertal archaeological record enables a close analysis of their technical knowledge structures and in turn grounds a provocative comparison with the technical cognition of modern humans.

Neandertals lived in Europe and Western Asia from about 300,000 years ago to about 40,000 years ago. They were anatomically very similar to the *Homo sapiens* who lived in Africa at the same time and who were the ancestors of modern humans. Neandertals did possess features that had evolved over the roughly 500,000 years during which the two groups had been isolated from one another, including features related to body build and cranio/facial anatomy. But did these differences include cognitive differences? This question underpins a perennial debate in paleoanthropology concerning the "status" of Neandertals, a debate that all too often has been poorly grounded (Botha, 2020; Wynn et al., 2016). Archaeological evidence of Neandertals consists of hundreds of known sites and scores of well-excavated sites. There is an especially rich record of Neandertal stone tools and archaeologists know a great deal about Neandertal flint knapping. Here, we focus on one very informative example, Marjorie's Core from Maastricht-Belvedere in the Netherlands (Schlanger, 1996).

Archaeologists at the University of Leiden excavated the open site of Maastricht-Belvedere in the 1980s and early 1990s (Roebroeks, 1988). Lithic remains included sets of flakes from Levallois cores, and analysts (including Marjorie) were able to refit the flakes into the original core mass. This refitting enabled Nathan Schlanger to describe the sequence of actions and decisions made by the original knapper, that is, a *chaîne opératoire*. The knapper followed a procedure that archaeologists have labeled "recurrent Levallois" in which the knapper produced a series of "predetermined" large flakes from a single prepared core. Predetermination is a misleading term. There was no need for the knapper to foresee a specific result, but the procedure did allow him or her to pursue the goal of producing large, flat flakes. The key to Levallois technique is the production of an asymmetrical prepared core with a deep convex base and shallower convexity above that acts as a production surface, the surface from which the knapper removed a large flake or flakes (see Fig. 7, which labels the important features of Levallois cores).

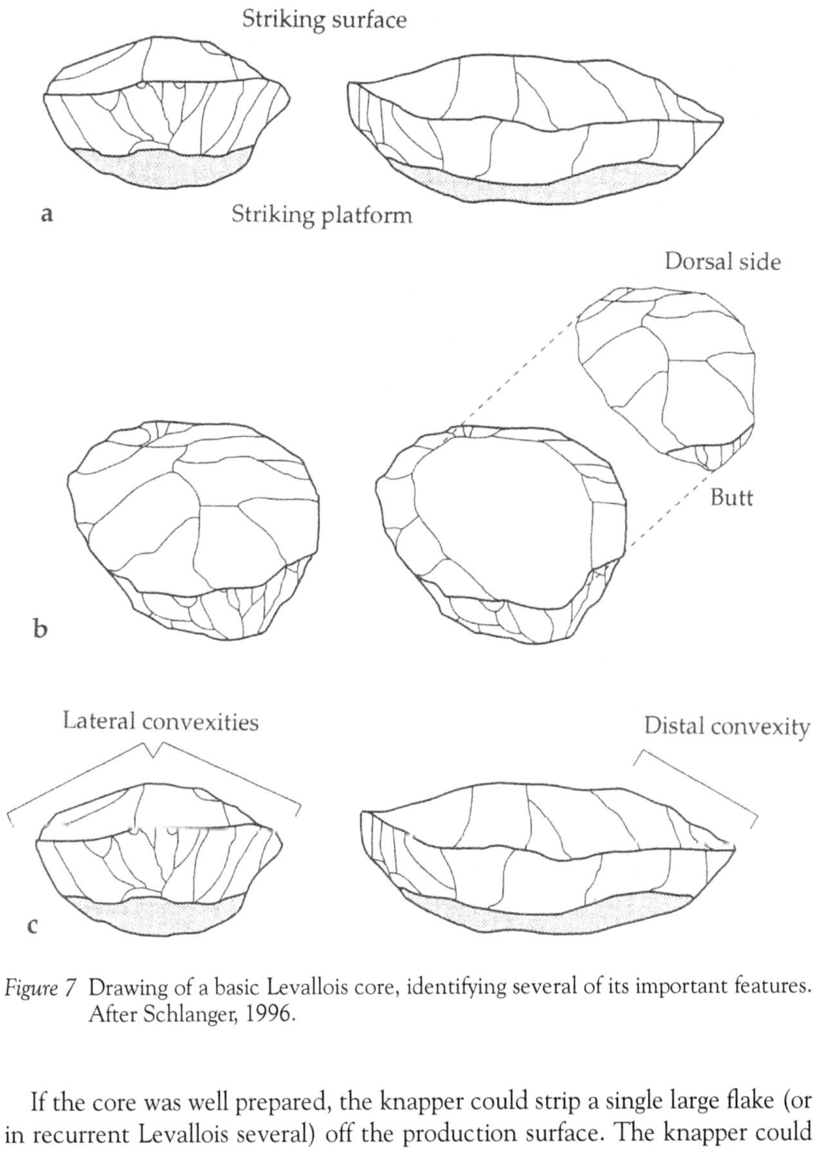

Figure 7 Drawing of a basic Levallois core, identifying several of its important features. After Schlanger, 1996.

If the core was well prepared, the knapper could strip a single large flake (or in recurrent Levallois several) off the production surface. The knapper could then reprepare the production surface and try again, which is what the knapper of Marjorie's Core did six times.

Fig. 8 presents Schlanger's summary of the sequence of discrete steps followed by the knapper.

It begins at the top with Phase 2 because the knapper initially prepared the core off site, perhaps at a quarry. The Arabic numbers identify the sequence of individual flake removals. Fig. 9 presents Phase 4 in more detail. We have added letters (x, y, z) to designate important features that guided the procedure.

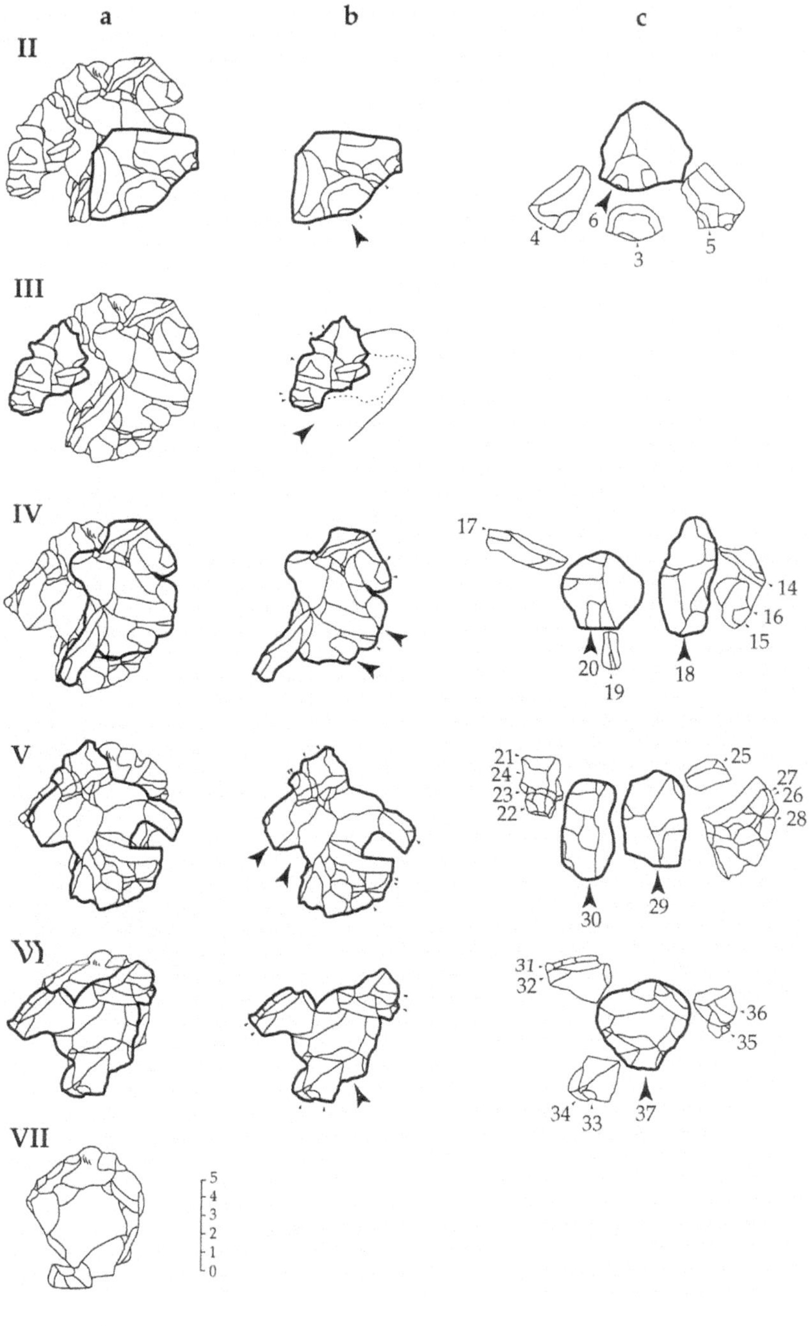

Figure 8 The sequence of steps Schlanger identified for Margorie's core. After Schlanger, 1996.

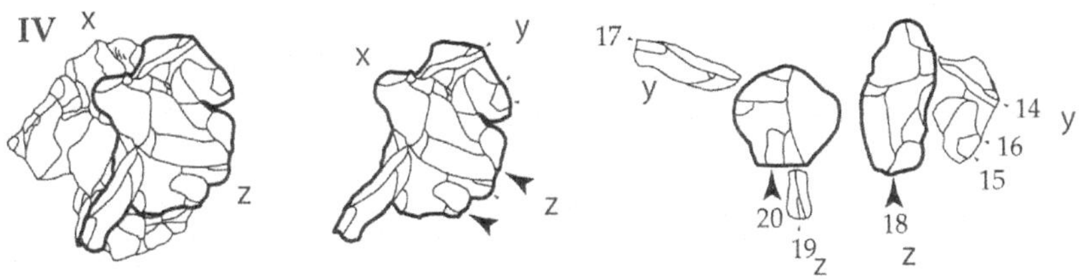

Figure 9 Step IV in the Marjorie's core reduction sequence.

Schlanger's *chaîne opératoire* enables us to identify components of the knapper's knowledge structure:

(1) After judging Phase 3 to be complete, the knapper identified a new distal convexity (X), which would be opposite the striking platform (Z). In the parlance of expert cognition, the distal convexity acted as a cue.
(2) The knapper prepared the lateral convexities (Y) by removing flakes 14 through 17. These convexities would ultimately guide the force along the production surface during the primary flake removal. At least two cues are evident in this step: one guiding the lateral convexities per se and one governing the overall configuration of the production surface.
(3) The knapper prepared the striking platform (Z). The angle between the striking and the production surface and the shape of the striking platform are critical variables in directing the force of the subsequent blow. Here again, the knapper responded to visual cues.
(4) The knapper struck off flake #18, which was a larger, targeted Levallois flake.
(5) He or she examined the core and saw that flake #18 had not exhausted the potential of this production surface and struck off a small flake (#19) to adjust the platform.
(6) He or she then struck off flake #20.
(7) The knapper then rotated the core 90° so that a lateral convexity became the distal convexity for the next phase.

From the perspective of expert cognition, the knapper of Marjorie's core used a knowledge structure that included at least seven different cues:

(1) Distal convexity
(2) Production surface
    (a) Lateral convexities
    (b) Location of striking platform
(3) Striking platform
    (a) Location of distal convexity
    (b) Angle with production surface

(c) Shape
(d) Ideal point of percussion

Schlanger's analysis of the Marjorie's core *chaîne opératoire* warrants several conclusions about Neandertal technical cognition. The sequence of phases indicates that the knapper followed the same strategy for each phase, guided by a recurring set of visuospatial cues and at least one declarative rule (rotate core 90° at completion of a step). In the terminology of expert cognition, this strategy reflects a well-established knowledge structure that facilitated rapid access to task relevant information stored in long-term memory, including motor procedures and techniques for managing core volume. Even though the analysis identified only a few of the total cues that must have been involved, it is still possible to identify features of the organization of the knowledge structure itself. First, it was hierarchical; some cues were components of higher level cues. The cue "production surface" elicited the cues "distal convexity," "lateral convexity," "platform position," and so forth. Each of these cues in turn elicited more specific cues consisting of angles, surfaces, ridges, and other visuospatial features inherent in stone knapping. Second, cues clearly changed according to their role in the procedure. What was a lateral convexity in one phase became a distal convexity in the next. Such flexibility is one of the hallmarks of expert performance. Finally, the phases of reduction were not independent of one another. The knapper conceived of a sequence of phases in order to maximize productivity of the core; while completing one phase, he or she looked forward to the next, an ability powered by the working memory component of expertise (Wynn & Coolidge, 2010a).

Actualistic studies of stone knapping corroborate Schlanger's analysis. Modern knappers generally agree that Levallois is one the most difficult procedures to master. Managing a core volume in this way requires familiarity with many, many small-scale challenges in the control of trimming, and the haptic/motor resources to deliver the requisite blows. Mastery of Levallois requires hundreds, perhaps even thousands, of repetitions, and few modern knappers are as adept as the knapper of Marjorie's core.

When we compare Levallois knowledge structures to those of modern handtool technology, a provocative conclusion becomes apparent: Neandertal and modern technical cognition are effectively indistinguishable. This does not mean that there were no differences between Neandertals and modern humans, but it does mean there were no obvious differences in how Neandertals and modern humans thought about and used tools. Indeed, it is possible to recognize expert knowledge structures back to the time of *Homo erectus*, at least (Alperson-Afil et al., 2020). About the only apparent difference is the sheer size of the knowledge chunks held in long-term memory. Technical expertise as described here is a very old strategy in hominin adaptations. Grounding an account in formal theories of expert performance allows us to stipulate which components must have evolved and perhaps the contexts in which this happened.

8 Spatial Cognition

In April 1916, Ernest Shackleton and four companions sailed a 20 ft (6.1 m) lifeboat from Elephant Island in Antarctica to South Georgia Island—830 nautical miles (1,500 km) across the stormiest seas on earth. It was an astonishing feat of seamanship and navigation and is justly celebrated in the annals of exploration. But Shackleton's feat was not unique. Micronesian sailors sail their outrigger canoes over the horizon to reach tiny atolls whose highest visible feature is a palm tree, all without a compass or a map. They can do this at night and in bad weather [and, anecdotally, after an evening of heavy drinking (Gladwin, 1970)]. We humans are very good at finding ourselves and moving in space. Unlike many birds, hominins do not have instinctive navigational abilities, so how are we able to move about in space so effectively? As is so often the case in human cognitive evolution, our spatial abilities rely on a combination of neurocognitive abilities and technical knowledge structures.

Modern humans use two different strategies to navigate (the preferred term is wayfinding)—route following and survey knowledge—and the two tap into different cognitive abilities. In route following, an individual traverses a series of segments defined by landmarks, for example, "drive until you come to a traffic signal, turn left and drive to the McDonald's, then turn right." This tactic relies on long-term sequential memory and working memory and is especially effective in well-known areas. Survey knowledge, on the other hand, relies on a person's ability to place himself or herself and a goal in the context of an external, permanent spatial framework. This could be latitude and longitude (Shackleton's) or some other system (Micronesian sailors use a system of celestial navigation). Cognitive requirements for survey knowledge fall in the domain of spatial perception and cognition, including one's ability in allocentric perception, which is the ability to imagine perspectives not centered on self (ego).

In addition to long-term memory, working memory, and allocentric perception, human wayfinding relies on knowledge structures similar to those in technical cognition, and these knowledge structures include embodied and artifactual components. Shackleton and his navigator, Frank Worseley, had learned a sophisticated survey system that could situate themselves and their goal in space and provide a route between them. Technology (sextant and an

DOI: 10.4324/9781003014485-10

accurate time piece) enabled them to find their position and maintain their course, something they could not have done without a technical extension. Micronesian sailors also rely on a knowledge structure, but one based on star positions and a learned system of dead reckoning known as "etak," in which they track imaginary reference islands moving across the star field. They also use their canoes to feel—literally through the seat of their pants—the action of waves and currents and the effects of shallowing and deepening water. Thus, the canoe itself becomes a component of the knowledge structure. As in technical cognition, wayfinding is an expert system learned via apprenticeship.

Every lobe of the brain comes into play during spatial cognition. The occipital lobes take in visual information and extract basic patterns, passing these visual percepts forward for higher level processing. There are two streams of visual processing. One is a ventral stream that passes information to the temporal lobes and processes shapes. The second is a dorsal stream that passes information to the parietal lobes that process more sophisticated spatial relations, including image manipulation. Situated beneath and internal to the temporal lobes is the hippocampus, whose posterior portion stores spatial representations and passes information to the medial gyrus of the temporal lobe for processing. In a famous study, Maguire et al. (2000) found that the posterior hippocampus of London taxi drivers was significantly larger than that of controls. London taxi drivers must pass a test of "The Knowledge," which includes the locations of all addresses in Central London (within a six-mile radius of Charing Cross) and optimal routes between them—25,000 separate streets. The parietal lobes process not only basic relations such as left-right and up-down but also more sophisticated relations such as those required in allocentric perception and other forms of visuospatial image transformation. The frontal lobes come into play when the brain applies motor resources in the manipulation of images and when the episodic buffer of working memory accesses visuospatial information.

Archaeologists have grounded discussions of spatial cognition in several different theories. In the 1970s and 1980s, Wynn interpreted stone tools using the genetic epistemology of Jean Piaget (see earlier discussion on page 23). This developmental theory had paid close attention to children's spatial thinking and provided Wynn with specific attributes to apply to stone tools. In the 1990s, evolutionary psychologist Irwin Silverman developed a hunter-gatherer theory for human spatial cognition that suggested that "space constancy," a version of allocentric perception, evolved as an aid to wayfinding. In the 1990s and 2000s, Derek Hodgson (2000, 2009) applied neurocognitive concepts of visual processing to the record of early stone tools and to the development of depiction. About the same time, Wynn (2002) turned to cognitive neuroscience as a more powerful theory for understanding the record of symmetry in stone tools. More recent works by Lycett (Key & Lycett, 2017) and Stout et al. (2015) have also addressed symmetry from a neurocognitive perspective, while Moore (Moore & Perston, 2016) has taken a more conservative approach that eschews the need for internal representations and focuses on the internal dynamics of stone knapping.

As always, archaeologists' access to relevant behaviors is limited by the nature of the archaeological record. To study wayfinding, for example, there would need to be traces of individuals and groups moving across landscapes. This in turn requires multiple locales visited by the same person or group. Such evidence might exist for recent time periods in well-studied areas, but it is almost unknown for the Palaeolithic. By identifying sources of raw material, Palaeolithic specialists can see how artifacts moved across a landscape, but without access to the agents themselves, this movement is only weakly indicative of wayfinding. Some large-scale events implicate wayfinding abilities. The colonization of the Sahul (Australia/New Guinea) is an excellent example (Davidson, 2010; Davidson & Noble, 1992). People had to make the journey over the horizon in watercraft of some kind. This would have been difficult to accomplish without some external framework of survey knowledge, though a simple rising sun-setting sun directionality would have sufficed (the Sahul is a big target). Material aids to wayfinding could be very informative, but only if reliably identified. Middle Stone Age (MSA) people in South Africa, for example, made shell beads that they strung together. This could have been a means of dead reckoning that used the beads to keep track of paces, as Klint Janulis has argued (Wynn et al., 2017). Of course, the beads might instead have been ornaments that lacked any wayfinding function; indeed, without any other indication of wayfinding, the ornament hypothesis is the more parsimonious of the two.

Most archaeologists who study spatial cognition focus on stone tools. To make a stone tool, the knapper must organize actions on the spatial field of the artifact and this organization reflects his or her understanding of spatial relations. This is not as limiting as it might seem. Most spatial cognition employed in wayfinding has parallels in the smaller scale manipulation of objects. For example, reliance on an external frame in survey knowledge has parallels in the use of allocentric reference frames in stone knapping.

The Boxgrove Handaxes and Allocentric Perception

Boxgrove is a 500,000-year-old archaeological landscape in southern Britain near the coast of the English Channel. Here, for a brief period of between 20 and 80 years, a drop in the interglacial (ISO 13) high sea levels exposed a locale of low relief bordered to the north by a chalk cliff from which nodules of high-quality gray flint eroded. Based on meticulous excavation at several sites, and subsequent analysis, the archaeology of Boxgrove has provided an extensive picture of the daily life of *Homo heidelbergensis* (Roberts & Parfitt, 1999). Most famous are the handaxes.

Fig. 10 is photo of three of the several hundred handaxes excavated at Boxgrove. The pristine preservation of the landscape at Boxgrove yielded not only handaxes but also several groups of trimming flakes produced by the manufacture of individual handaxes, enabling archaeologists to identify most of the procedures that made up the knappers' expert knowledge structures. These

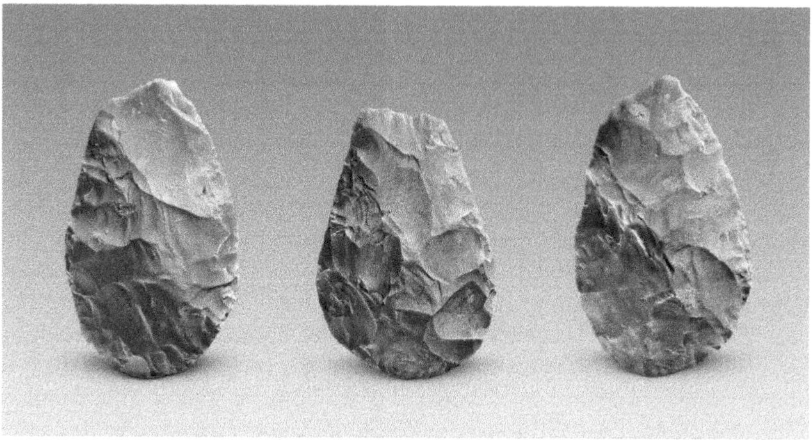

Figure 10 Boxgrove handaxes. The rightmost is 15 × 8.9 cm.

knappers were especially adept at finishing the artifacts, a task that included striking long "thinning" flakes that extended across much of the breadth of the artifact and reduced the central thickness of the tool. Almost all the hundreds of handaxes are remarkably similar in size and shape, indicating that a tight community norm guided the knappers. However, it is also possible to identify idiosyncratic techniques and patterns that could identify individual knappers. An overarching goal governed all the knappers—produce an artifact with an excellent three-dimensional symmetry. It is this ability that reveals something important about their spatial cognition.

Symmetry is a common feature of living organisms and inanimate objects such as crystals, but it is not a feature of flint nodules or indeed of most knappable rock types. The knappers had to impose this form on the artifacts. A small minority of archaeologists think that the symmetries were unintended consequences of a flaking procedure (e.g., Davidson & Noble, 1993), but most scholars consider handaxe symmetries to have been intended. And imposition of symmetry informs us about aspects of spatial cognition. Derek Hodgson (2009, 2015) has emphasized the role of the visual processing system in the detection and appreciation of symmetry. Symmetry is an example of a "good Gestalt"—a regular form that by itself elicits pleasure. The vertebrate visual cortex has cell groups that are attuned to symmetrical patterns in the visual field, especially vertical or horizontal bilateral symmetries. When these cell groups activate, they send neural impulses forward in the brain to cells in the pleasure/reward system. There are good evolutionary reasons for this. Food (e.g., fruit) and danger (e.g., lions) have symmetrical features, and rapid detection had a selective payoff. Similarly, a symmetrical object, including a tool, is more pleasing to the eye than an amorphous lump. Thus, when early hominins began producing large cutting tools about

2 million years ago, some of those tools were more pleasing to look at. However, to *make* such pleasing forms, something in addition to symmetry-sensitive visual cell groups was needed. Stone knapping is a motor activity guided by the spatial resources of the dorsal processing stream (Stout et al., 2000). Symmetry is a salient shape detected by the ventral processing stream. In order to produce a symmetrical stone tool, the knapper had to coordinate these separate streams (Wynn, 2002). This required developments in the central processing resources of visuo-spatial working memory (Wynn & Coolidge, 2016). Thus, the bilateral symmetry of early handaxes (>1 million years old) attests to the evolution of spatial cognitive abilities beyond the abilities of apes.

The Boxgrove handaxes required yet another development in spatial cognition—the ability to imagine a viewpoint different from that of ego (the knapper's visual field) (Wynn, 2010). If one were to take a diamond-edged saw and cut through a Boxgrove handaxe at any angle, it would reveal a regular, symmetrical cross-section. The artifacts are symmetrical in three dimensions. The challenge to producing such regular cross-sections is that the knapper could not see them directly; he or she had to imagine them. The ability to imagine nonego-centered viewpoints is known as allocentric perception. It is one of the prerequisites for survey knowledge and a Euclidean understanding of space in which points have permanent, invariant positions in relation to one another.

The simple conclusion to this bit of analysis is one of the more robust in evolutionary cognitive archaeology. Because the Boxgrove hominins used allocentric perception in making their handaxes, we know that they had the ability to imagine and manipulate images. Both these abilities are necessary for constructing an external reference frame for use in survey knowledge. Moreover, allocentric perception is how many modern people think about space. Did *Homo heidelbergensis* have fully modern spatial cognition? Maybe. What are missing from the archaeological record, or least left no trace, are any extended artifactual resources that might have aided wayfinding. There are no maps or measuring devices of any kind at Boxgrove. Without them, feats such as those performed by Micronesian sailors or Ernest Shackleton would have been impossible. Nevertheless, the evidence from the Boxgrove handaxes suggests that human spatial cognition evolved a very long time ago, before *Homo sapiens* appeared on the evolutionary stage.

9 Social Cognition

As primates, humans are social animals. We live in groups year-round and rely on group efforts to achieve most of our wants and goals. As the ubiquity of social media in our current lives attests, we spend a significant proportion of daily time maintaining our social relationships. Not surprisingly, we are very good at it, or at least we think we are. Any account of human cognitive evolution must take social thinking into account. The archaeology of social cognition is one of the more challenging branches of evolutionary cognitive archaeology.

Social psychology is a vast subfield of psychology that has largely been untapped by evolutionary scholars. Instead, scholars interested in the evolution of social cognition have relied primarily on comparative psychology, study of nonhuman primates in particular, and evolutionary psychology, which has a keen interest in social cognition. The two subfields of psychological science approach human evolution rather differently. Comparative psychology relies on interpolation. If most anthropoid primates demonstrate a particular cognitive ability and modern humans demonstrate an enhanced version of that ability, then it is reasonable to conclude that this cognitive difference arose in the human evolutionary past. For example, all modern people easily pass a mirror recognition test (Povenelli, 1987), but most other anthropoids fail (chimpanzees are the occasional exception). Thus, at some point in human evolution, our hominin ancestors acquired enhanced abilities in self-definition and recognition. Evolutionary psychologists rely primarily on reverse engineering. Through well-designed experiments they isolate psychological adaptations that underpin certain behaviors. David Buss, as noted earlier, famously documented a perceptual bias in males for features in females associated with fecundity; mating is of course a primary component of social behavior, and there would be a definite advantage to quickly identifying fecund members of the opposite sex (Buss, 2003). Leda Cosmides identified another peculiarity of human social thinking—the ability to detect cheaters in social situations (Cosmides, 1989). Neither comparative psychology nor evolutionary psychology provides much insight into the timing, or even the sequence of these developments.

Primates are unusual, though not unique, among mammals because most primates incorporate adult males into their permanent social groups. Because we are primates and thus regularly deal with adult males, this seems quite

DOI: 10.4324/9781003014485-11

normal. But adult males present social problems. For mammals, at least, they tend to be larger and more aggressive. And they fight more, especially over resources and females. Adult females compete, too, but because they also must nurture offspring their energy budgets do not allow similar increases in size and aggressiveness. As a consequence, primate social lives are very complex, and primates have evolved an array of adaptations tied to this social complexity. Indeed, much of the focus of evolutionary psychology has been on cognitive adaptations to complex social lives. Here, we list just a few of the adaptations that primates, as a group, have evolved (Jolly, 1985; Tomasello & Call, 1997):

- Facial mobility and recognition: The anthropoid primates (monkeys, apes, and humans) have fine muscle control over their faces and extensive cell groups in the fusiform gyrus for detecting faces and facial expressions, which are important clues to others' moods.
- Polyadic monitoring: Most mammals interact socially via dyadic relationships—two individuals interacting. Primates, especially anthropoids, monitor polyadic (multiple) relations. For example, they attend to how their actions toward individual A will affect their relationship to individual B.
- Affective bonding: Primates form affective bonds with individuals other than their mothers. This is an avenue to alliance formation.
- Alliance formation: Primates form alliances for mutual benefit of members.
- Tactical deception: Primates deceive other individuals in order to acquire beneficial resources or to avoid aggression.

Primate cognition has evolved to be especially good at group life. Indeed, in the 1980s, Richard Byrne and Andrew Whiten, drawing on earlier work by Humphrey (1976) and Jolly (1985), formulated and defended the Machiavellian hypothesis, which argued that primate intelligence evolved to negotiate the complexities of social group life (Byrne & Whiten, 1988). They emphasized tactical deception and other mechanisms of social manipulation. Also in the 1980s, evolutionary psychologist Leda Cosmides (1989) identified a human ability to detect social cheaters and suggested that this was an important cognitive adaption that arose during human evolution. But there is more to primate social life than competition.

In 1990s, Robin Dunbar et al. proposed an alternative social model—they labeled the Social Brain Hypothesis (SBH) (Dunbar et al., 2010, 2014). The hypothesis is based on a provocative correlation. The relative neocortex size (neocortex/overall brain size) of primate species varied according to their average social group size; primates who lived in larger face-to-face social groups had larger neocortices. Dunbar argued that maintaining social bonds between individuals was more challenging in larger groups and that grooming, vocal communication, and ultimately language evolved to solve this challenge to social success. Advocates of the SBH have identified other cognitive abilities that they believe evolved in support of social cognition, including Theory of Mind (ToM), which is the ability to imagine what another individual is thinking.

A related ability is social learning, which is learning from observing the actions of another and, more provocatively, through teaching.

Documenting social cognition is a difficult challenge for archaeologists. The difficulty, identified by Hawkes in his ladder of inference, is that social behaviors do not themselves preserve in archaeological remains. If one wants to study social cognition, one must first make an inference from a pattern of material remains to the social action responsible. This adds an additional link to the chain of inferences, a link that must be appropriately grounded and warranted. Inferences to social actions are especially prone to equifinality. Hawkes's example is worth repeating. Perhaps the most commonly encountered pattern of architecture in the archaeological record is a circular hut 4–5 m in diameter. Hunting and gathering bands often made them; Neolithic agriculturalists made them; and Iron Age peasants made them. Alone, these huts cannot distinguish between these very different forms of social organization.

Archaeologists interested in social cognition have a limited range of potentially informative evidence. Most informative, despite equifinality, is settlement pattern, which includes sizes and locations of features (e.g., hearths), structures, and sites. Because of the sliding scale of preservation, such evidence is mostly available for very recent time periods, after 10,000 years ago. Ideational cognitive archaeologists find such evidence useful; interpretations of the ideational system behind the Neolithic/Bronze Age monument of Stonehenge are excellent examples (Parker Pearson, 2012). For most of human evolution, however, hominin settlement pattern consisted of residential and activity sites of limited occupational duration, almost always disturbed by erosion or subsequent hominin occupation. Such evidence is a challenge, but it is not entirely mute. For example, Neandertals and the modern humans who followed them often occupied the same rock-shelters in the Perigord region of southwestern France (Gamble, 1999). The Neandertal remains typically cover a small area of perhaps 35–100 m^2, often entirely within the shelter. Modern human remains are typically far more extensive (within a shorter time frame) and extend laterally well beyond the confines of the shelter. What does this distinction in residential area suggest? Most specialists agree that the average face-to-face residential units of Neandertals, and modern humans must have been quite different in size. Larger face-to-face groups present social challenges not present in smaller groups and may have selected for cognitive abilities unneeded by Neandertals (Wynn & Coolidge, 2012).

Artifacts themselves provide clues to social life. Evidence for long distance social contacts is one example. In late Palaeolithic sites, archaeologists occasionally recover items whose origin lay hundreds of kilometers away. Most often, these are ornaments of one kind or another, though tools of high-quality raw material occasionally moved equally far. This is evidence for long range social contact and perhaps even trade (which is hard to demonstrate without actual evidence of exchange). Equifinality rears its ugly head here as well; there are multiple social models for moving artifacts long distances, but all share a significant factor—the ability to interact with strangers and remote acquaintances

(Belfer-Cohen & Hovers, 2020). Several cognitive abilities identified by evolutionary psychologists, such as cheater detection (Cosmides, 1989) and "market pricing" (Fiske, 2004) may well have evolved as aids to dealing with strangers. Archaeological evidence for such long-range interactions is sparse until late in the Palaeolithic, and they may have been one of the advantages that modern humans had over Neandertals.

The emergence of artifact styles is another potential window onto social cognition. Archaeologists use the term style in several different ways. Perhaps most commonly, they use style to refer to repetitive patterns that people in the past chose to impose on their artifacts. These were conscious expressions of personal or group standards or norms, as in "I [person X] always notch projectile points this way," or "We [people X] always decorate pots this way." Such imposed styles are ubiquitous in modern culture and often act as emblems of group identity. There is a second form of style that James Sackett (1982) labeled "isochrestic." Isochrestic styles result from unconscious adherence to a way of doing things. If one learns a technical procedure from a mentor, the choices one learns to make will often be somewhat arbitrary; other choices might work equally well, but one only learns a single option. The combination of these choices produces a repeated pattern in material culture, and this pattern can "stand for" the artisan, that is, others can recognize the artisan's work. Finally, archaeologists often use the term style for purely analytical classes of artifacts associated with a place or a time period, such as Bell Beakers or Linearbandkeramik (Whittle, 1996). The topic of style in archaeology is reminiscent of the topic of typology, and many of the same methodological issues arise. Here, we are interested in what style can reveal about social interaction, and thus, the first two uses are most relevant (emblematic and isochrestic). Cognitively, adherence to emblematic stylistic standards implies the active recognition of community norms (also known as normative behavior), whereas isochrestic style requires no such active adherence; it simply emerges from the pedagogical system. Distinguishing between the two is tricky; both produce repetitive artifact forms.

Recently, for example, Ceri Shipton and Mark White have argued that normativity was a component of social cognition 500,000 years ago in Britain (Shipton & White, 2020). They warranted this conclusion via an analysis of shape variability in handaxes (analysis of handaxe shape variability is a motif running through the last 60 years of Palaeolithic archaeology). They used a sophisticated morphometric imaging system and analyzed the variability in form using principle component analysis. They concluded that the range of form at sites such as Boxgrove is too narrow to represent isochrestic style alone (they do not use the term) and that the hominin knappers must have attended to a community-wide norm.

Shipton and White include reference to "learning chains," and the subject of social learning is yet another way to document social interaction. There is an extensive literature on social learning in cognitive psychology and primatology and also detailed ethnographic accounts from anthropology. In addition, social learning is accessible to experimental protocols and statistical analyses. This wealth of potential grounding theories and methodological approaches provides ECA with a toolkit with which to approach one variety of social interaction. Of course, most social learning was dyadic—one individual learning from another. Thus, studies of the evolution of social learning address only a very narrow range of social interactions. Not surprisingly, most ECA applications have tackled what varieties of social learning are implied by various kinds of lithic technology. For example, Morgan et al. (2015) used an experimental protocol in which novices learned to knap basic Oldowan-like stone tools and then tried to transfer their knowledge to a new "generation" of novice knappers using a variety of controlled learning style, including imitation and linguistic instruction. In a more ambitious discussion, Gärdenfors and Högberg (Gärdenfors & Högberg, 2017) define a taxonomy of varieties of teaching, including intentional evaluative feedback, drawing attention, demonstrating, communicating concepts, and explaining relations between concepts. They then turned to the Palaeolithic record and tried to identify points in the Palaeolithic sequence when each of these teaching styles became necessary, based on the complexity of the technical procedures. For example, they argue that "learning the late Acheulean hand-axe technology [e.g., at sites such as Boxgrove—TW] is made possible by the teacher, who assists the learner in understanding the structure of the sub-goals by teaching how to perceive patterns" (Gädenfors & Högberg, 2017, p. 194). This technology, they argue, could not be learned by imitation alone. The nature of teaching might seem a narrow social domain with limited implications for cognitive evolution, but it is also a window on other domains, such as language and ToM.

Cole's Identity Model and Theory of Mind

Perhaps, the most thorough application of ToM to the archaeological record is that of James Cole (2014, 2017). Beginning in the 1990s, as we mentioned earlier, Robin Dunbar et al. developed the Social Brain Hypothesis for the evolution of primate cognition that emphasized the establishment and maintenance of social relationships. Although they focused on neocortex size and social group size, they also identified ToM in general, and orders of intentionality in particular, as being likely components of increasingly powerful social cognition. First-order intentionality is self-awareness ("I know"); second order is awareness that one has a mind and that another individual has a different mind ("I know that you know"); third order is awareness that another is aware that you are aware ("I know that you know that I know"); and so on. Humans are quite good at this kind of thing; it is the basis of our love of gossip and social media, for example. Most people can handle fifth-order intentionality if pressed, and a few can do better, with seven apparently maxing out the human range.

Dunbar et al. attempted to correlate order of intentionality with frontal lobe size (Dunbar, 1993, 1998) and used hominin endocasts as evidence. Cole set out to document the evolution of orders of intentionality using the Palaeolithic archaeological record. If you recall from our earlier discussion, accessing social cognition through material remains requires an additional link in the chain of inference, an inference about social interaction. To ground this inference, Cole turned to the psychological literature on identity formation. Here, he found a robust theory of personal identity construction that emphasized the role of others and groups in defining one's self-identity and which articulated easily with levels of intentionality. *Individual identity*, an awareness of self (ego), requires first-order intentionality; *external identity* is an awareness that another has an opinion about ego and requires second-order intentionality; in *manipulated individual identity*, ego alters the identity that another sees, and this requires third-order intentionality; for *collective identity*, ego manipulates identity to conform to a community norm and employs fourth-order intentionality. Of course, none of this preserves directly in the archaeological record. But here, Cole made a clever choice. He turned to the archaeological and anthropological literature on the role of material culture in structuring and mediating social relations. By combining these two otherwise separate theories of social action, he was able to develop a workable model in which material culture acts to help create and mediate identities based on higher order intentionalities. For example, when hominins began to alter the form of artifacts in nonfunctional ways, it implies that they took into account what others could see and manipulated how others saw ego. This is third-order intentionality. Later, when hominins clearly adhered to community-wide standards, this implicated fourth-order and perhaps fifth-order intentionality.

We find Cole's model to be especially persuasive because he has been explicit about his theoretical grounding (identity theory; material-social construction) and how artifacts warrant inferences about intentionality. In other words, he makes all the components of a cognitive interpretation explicit. This in turn opens it up to constructive discussion and disagreement. Shipton and White (2020), noted earlier, make a strong argument for normativity (community standards) as early as 500,000 years ago. In Cole's scheme, this is *prima facie* evidence for fourth-order intentionality. Orders of intentionality and ToM also have implications for other components of cognition. There is, for example, a clear role of working memory in orders of intentionality (Wynn & Coolidge, 2009) and Cole's argument for identity tracks other indications of working memory capacity nicely. ToM also plays a role in symbol use and language.

10 Art and Aesthetics

Art is a human universal. All people, everywhere, engage in artistic performances of one kind or another, and many consider artistic pursuits to be among the most meaningful human activities. Archaeologists, too, have a serious interest in art; indeed, Enlightenment Era antiquarians had an abiding interest in the recovery and identification of Classical Age statuary, mosaics, and architecture. Art is a natural target for cognitive archaeologists as well. The interpretation of prehistoric art is one of the central concerns of ideational cognitive archaeologists because it provides access to the belief systems of the artisans. Evolutionary cognitive archaeologists have been more circumspect in their approach to art, partly because the literature on the evolution of art is riddled with poorly grounded claims. Everyone, it would seem, knows art when they see it, and thus feel little need to ground their claims in careful reasoning. Art is an important form of human expression and communication, and its cognitive basis is an important component of the human mind. It is thus appropriate to study its evolution.

Art, however, is notoriously hard to define, making controlled studies of its cognitive basis tricky. What counts as art? Should we include architecture, for example, or automobiles, or terraced paddy fields? Some might limit art to "fine" art, available for admiration in museums or sale in galleries. Others would include craft, such as weaving, blacksmithing, and ceramics (most archaeologists would fall in this group). Drawing boundaries around art turns out to be a thankless task. In the late 1990s, neuroscientists and psychologists took up the challenge of describing how people think about art. However, rather than tackle "art," with all its social and cultural accoutrements, the brain sciences focused on the related domain of aesthetics—the perception and appreciation of beauty. Aesthetics differs from art in its narrower focus on phenomena that elicit emotional responses but also directs this focus at a broader range of phenomena, including responses to natural scenes (e.g., sunsets) and forms (e.g., faces). Neuroaesthetics is the interdisciplinary study of the neural underpinnings of aesthetic experience and utilizes the resources of experimental cognitive psychology and neuroimaging (Chatterjee, 2014; Leder & Nadal, 2014; Ramachandran & Hirstein, 1999; Zeki, 1999). Research in neuroaesthetics is now well-enough established that it can ground inferences using the archaeological record.

DOI: 10.4324/9781003014485-12

The first generalization from neuroaesthetics research is simple but important: there is no single neural network or group of neurons dedicated to aesthetic experience and active in no other. Instead, aesthetic experience draws on several overlapping neural networks that each evolved for other purposes. Neuroaestheticians differ slightly in how they parse these neural systems, but most identify three or four primary neural networks. Here, we will follow Chatterjee (2014), who identifies three: (1) sensorimotor, (2) emotion-evaluation, and (3) meaning-knowledge.

Sensorimotor processing includes the cell groups that receive input from the sense organs and perform the initial processing that transforms sensations into perceptions. Using vision as an example (it is the best understood), sensory data from the retinas travel to the occipital cortex via the optic chiasm for initial processing. There are built-in biases. For example, more cell groups react to vertical and horizontal line and edge orientation that to oblique lines. All sensations are not equal, and even at this primary level, some sensations elicit positive affect, that is pleasure, through activation of mu-opioid-producing cells (Hodgson, 2000, 2009, 2017). As we mentioned in the section on spatial cognition, the brain passes this upgraded visual information forward from the occipital lobes in two streams, a dorsal stream connected to the parietal lobes, and a ventral stream connected to the temporal lobes, the fusiform gyrus in particular, where the brain handles shape recognition. And here, too, the brain demonstrates bias toward some percepts over others. Helmut Leder and colleagues (Leder et al., 2004; Leder & Nadal, 2014) have identified what they have termed "implicit memory effects," which are salient visual effects that elicit pleasure, but which are pre-attentive, that is, they are effective without conscious attention. Four of these implicit effects are important in visual aesthetics. **Peak shift** is the exaggeration of patterns that elicit positive affect and is regularly exploited by artists in the modern world. Political cartoonists, for example, typically exaggerate facial features of familiar public figures. Such exaggerations can include size, shapes, and even color. Shapes that approach the ideal **prototype** for a class of perceptual phenomena also elicit pleasure. Symmetry is a good example. **Familiarity** is a related effect and encounters with familiar perceptual phenomena elicit greater positive affect than unfamiliar phenomena. Finally, visual perception responds positively to patterns that focus attention by **framing** phenomena toward the center of the visual field. All these effects are pre-attentive and thus occur without volition. This does not mean that the salient patterns are preprogrammed genetically, though some visual biases clearly are. Learning does play a role, especially in regard to familiarity and prototypicality.

A second neural network involved in aesthetic processing governs emotion and evaluation. One of the important differences between aesthetics and other domains of perception is the incorporation of evaluation and affect. We like something, or we dislike it, or it leaves us unmoved. This network incorporates both pre-attentive: "bottom-up" processing and "top-down" attentive resources. They generate a range of emotional responses from transcendence to repulsion (Brown et al., 2011). Neural resources that govern emotion are involved, such as the orbitofrontal cortex and anterior cingulate cortex, but the structure that appears to be the key component in appraisal itself is the anterior insula, which lies deep within the lateral sulcus. It evolved initially in support of gustatory taste; liking healthful foods and disliking unhealthful foods had a strong survival value. Over the course of mammalian evolution, the anterior insula came to be exapted for other forms of evaluation. Thus, aesthetic taste literally relies on resources that evolved for tasting food.

The final network engaged in aesthetic experience is meaning-knowledge. This is a vast neural network that includes all the top-down knowledge resources that people bring to aesthetic experience, including both performing and observing. These resources include implicit and explicit memories, autonoesis, and social cognition; how one experiences an aesthetic phenomenon can vary dramatically according to immediate physical and social context, and personal and social history. Autobiographical memory is especially important. Our personal experience with an aesthetic phenomenon has a profound effect on how we experience it in the present and if we revisit it in the future. We can learn to like and dislike. Moreover, our autobiographical milieu provides a wealth of symbolic and indexical meanings that have accrued to aesthetic experiences, to the extent that we find it quite natural to ask what an aesthetic product means, as if explicit meaning is inherent to all aesthetic phenomena. However, it needn't be. This erroneous assumption has led many archaeologists to make unwarranted claims about the past.

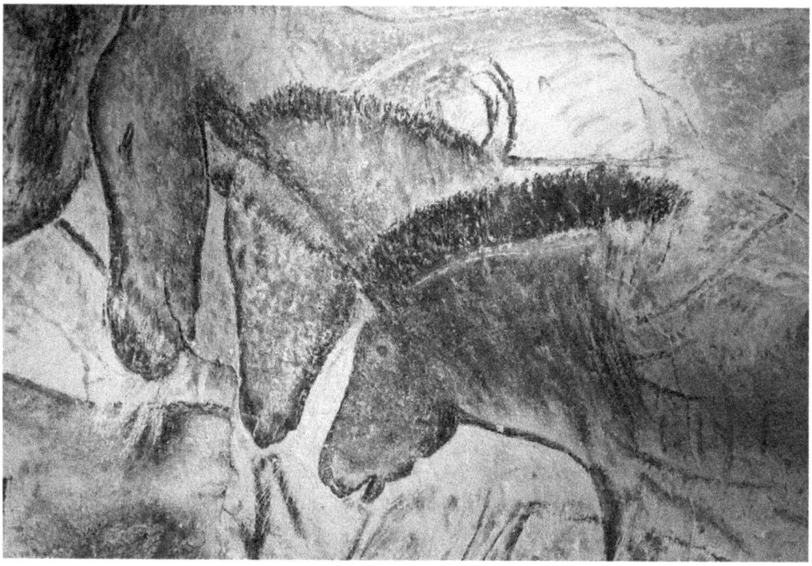

Figure 11 Paintings of rhinoceros in Chauvet Cave, ca. 39,000 BP. Claude Valette. CC BY-SA 4.0.

The establishment of neuroaesthetics as a vibrant field in cognitive science has provided archaeologists with a framework for addressing the perennially fractious topic of early art and decorative systems, especially Palaeolithic examples that antedate the appearance of the famous cave paintings of Western Europe.

There appears to be general agreement among archaeologists and art historians alike that these spectacular depictions of animals and geometric designs deserve the appellation of "art" in the modern sense and that all the components parsed by neuroaesthetics were in play, including a well-developed system of symbolic meaning. Unfortunately, there are no known antecedents for this tradition of cave art; it arrived fully developed in Europe about 40,000 years ago. No earlier, cruder versions exist. It is therefore necessary to look to other kinds of aesthetic productions. Because aesthetics is underpinned by several overlapping, but still functionally discrete neural networks, we cannot assume that aesthetic cognition evolved as a package; in the modern world, they do appear to be a unified aesthetic sensitivity, but this need not have been the case in the evolutionary past. For example, evidence for application of implicit visual effects does not require the presence of symbolic meaning.

The Blombos Engravings

Artifacts from the South African Middle Stone Age site of Blombos Cave have been touchstones in an archaeological debate about the emergence of modern behavior, art, and symbolism. Beginning in the 1990s, Christopher Henshilwood and colleagues excavated several provocative categories of artifacts that extended the time depth of aesthetic productions back to 77,000 years before present. Two categories of evidence have been the center of a spirited debate—shell beads and engraved pieces of ochre. The beads are shells of *Nassarius* sp. that are bright blue when fresh. People living at Blombos collected them from a nearby estuary, carefully punched a hole in each, and strung them on a cord of some sort. We know this because of a careful microscopic study

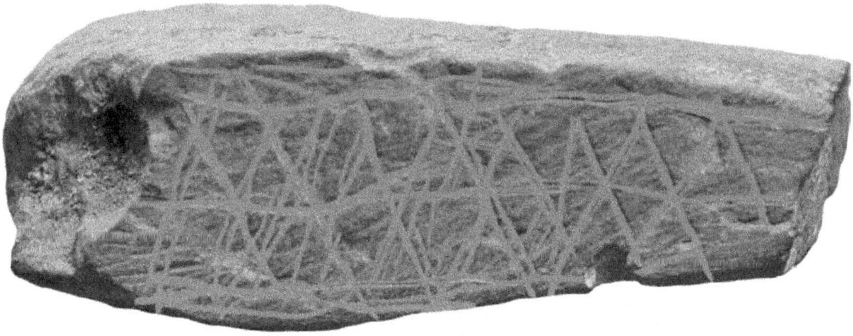

Figure 12 Blombos engraving on ground surface of a "pencil" of ochre, ca. 8 cm (Hodgson, 2014).

wear patterns done by archaeologist Francesco d'Errico (d'Errico et al., 2003, 2008). The engravings are perhaps more provocative from an aesthetic perspective. They are cross-hatched designs engraved into the surfaces of pieces of ochre, a mineral pigment.

The regularity and arrangement of the lines effectively eliminates any possibility that these were natural or random effects. Someone produced the design deliberately. Almost all participants in the debate agree on these descriptive facts. Interpretation has not been so agreeable. Henshilwood himself, working with d'Errico and others, argued that the beads and engravings were evidence of modern symbolic culture, including language and art (d'Errico et al., 2003, 2008; Henshilwood & Dubreuil, 2011). Many, indeed most, Palaeolithic specialists agreed and celebrated this breakthrough in understanding the origin of modern symbolism and art. But not everyone was convinced. As discussed earlier, linguist Rudolf Botha detected a serious logical flaw in the logic concerning language. But what about the suggestion that the engravings were solid evidence of art? This claim has been most effectively challenged by Derek Hodgson.

Hodgson (2014, 2017) argued that the cross-hatched engravings could be understood more parsimoniously as patterns that elicited pleasure via the visual processing system itself. He labels his hypothesis the Neurovisual Resonance hypothesis and has applied it not just to 77,000-year-old engravings, but to a selection of artifacts going back 1.7 million years to the advent of handaxes. Put simply, making geometric patterns is pleasurable in its own right. The patterns need not have had any symbolic message, or even shared meaning or value. Hodgson was able to account for the engravings, and much more, by invoking the sensorimotor component of aesthetic experience alone. Henshilwood and d'Errico made the unwarranted assumption that the symbolic meaning component of modern aesthetic cognition must also have been in play because in modern aesthetics it is indeed a package. But, as we have seen, and Hodgson masterfully documents, this needn't have been true in deep past. That Hodgson's hypothesis has also been a productive approach to much earlier hominin aesthetics makes it that much more powerful.

11 Symbolism and Language

Archaeologist John Robb (1998) noted, "Archaeologists probably disagree about symbols more than anything else they dig up" (p. 329). Ironically, he never offered a definition of symbols in his article entitled, *The Archaeology of Symbols*, although he wrote of their relationship to power, prestige, gender, political studies, cosmological reconstructions, and other constructs. Robb also argued that all archaeological cultural phenomena were symbolic, but again, he offered no further clarity for its definition and no further explanation for his claim that all cultural phenomena were symbolic. Interestingly, definitions of language are equally contentious. For example, there are heated debates over whether there were earlier or primitive versions of language, called protolanguage (Arbib & Bickerton, 2010), or whether language sprung up suddenly and "whole-cloth" (e.g., Bolhuis et al., 2014).

A common dictionary definition of a symbol is that it is the use of a sign or mark to represent some idea, object, or relationship. Frequently, definitions of a symbol include that it is an arbitrary referent (or not so arbitrary) for what it actually represents, there is no resemblance (or there may be) between the signifier and the signified, and it must be culturally learned or appear in a cultural context (mandatory).

Symbolism and language are not themselves discrete cognitive abilities, yet they have come to be closely associated with cognitive archaeology, to the degree that we feel compelled to provide a brief account in this introductory text. There are several reasons for this perception. The most important is the undeniable salience of symbolism and language in our daily lives, but there are also reasons embedded in the last 50 years of archaeological scholarship.

Modern life is immersed in symbols. There are the obvious explicitly symbolic systems of religion, art, music, and literature, some of which play out through extensive social institutions and provide frameworks for understanding our very existence. But there are also less obvious symbols that permeate almost everything we do: traffic signs, clothing, building décor, architecture, even the way we fix our hair and walk down the street. All have symbolic meaning of a sort. Other people regularly decode the meanings of the symbols we project, and thus, symbolic meaning is an indispensable component of our lives. This is true for all people, everywhere, and thus, understanding

DOI: 10.4324/9781003014485-13

semiotics—the formal term for the study of symbolic systems—is an important component of anthropology and archaeology. People in the past also immersed their lives in symbols and left ample evidence in the form of monuments, art, decorative systems, and the minutiae of daily life. Thus, understanding of the past requires an understanding of symbols. Indeed, symbols are the primary focus of ideational cognitive archaeology.

The investigation of symbolic systems has always posed problems for archaeologists; Hawkes, for example, placed it on the most difficult rung of his ladder of inference (see Chapter 2). Treatments have also varied according to theoretic fashion. The demise of materialist theory in the 1970s can be partly blamed on its inability to account adequately for symbolic behavior. This failure was impetus for the development of ideational cognitive archaeology as well as several other theoretical slants that today prevail in archaeological studies of the recent past (<10,000 BP). Palaeolithic specialists have been the major holdouts and continue to favor materialist and ecological interpretations. But even they have not avoided symbolism altogether. Instead of interpreting symbols, Palaeolithic specialists have focused on documenting a chronology for the initial appearance and subsequent development of symbolic behavior. For many, it has become a marker for modern behavior, a development that has proven controversial and perhaps even counterproductive.

As noted earlier, symbols are commonly defined as "something that stands for or suggests something else" and few would disagree that this is an adequate general definition for use in everyday academic discourse. But it is quite "lumpy," in the sense that it encompasses a variety of phenomena and is thus difficult to use if one is interested in evolution. Crucifixes are clearly symbols in this sense (standing for the passion of Christ), but so are footprints (standing for the individual who made them), and so are photographs. However, these "symbols" differ from one another in terms of both how the "standing for" happens and the nature of the information delivered. Indeed, these differences are so significant and subtle that they are the focus of an entire academic discipline—semiotics. Semioticians use the term "sign" rather than symbol for the general category of "things that stand for something else." They have devised various schemes for cataloguing and explaining the variety of signs. In these contexts, "symbol" is a more narrowly delimited variety of sign. Perhaps, the two most influential semiotic catalogues are those of Swiss linguist Ferdinand de Saussure (1857–1913) and American philosopher Charles Sanders Peirce (1939–1914) (Stanford Encyclopedia of Philosophy 2010). As Peirce's scheme is currently more in vogue and has powered several provocative archaeological treatments, we turn to it.

Peirce distinguishes between the sign, the object it stands for, and the "interpretant," which is the sign-object relation, that is, how the sign delivers the reference to the object. Peirce's scheme then distinguishes between three major varieties in the way that the interpretant links the sign to the object: icons, indexes, and symbols. **Icons** link the sign to the object through physical resemblance, most typically visual resemblance. A drawing of a deer stands for a deer, and thus is an icon, and the interpretant is iconic reference. An **index** links a sign to its object by extension, connection, or association. A foot made the footprint, which is thus an extension of the foot, and can therefore refer to it. The interpretant is indexical reference. **Symbols** link to their objects through convention and are often arbitrary. Readers of English agree (convention) that "DEER" stands for a word and that the word stands for a particular animal. "DEER" does not resemble a deer, nor is it an extension of a deer. The interpretant is arbitrary and conventional. Signs can exploit more than one interpretant. The crucifix is an excellent example. It is iconic via an image of a crucified man; it is indexical via the cross's extension as an instrument of execution; and it is symbolic via the conventional, arbitrary meanings Christianity has assigned to it. Without access to the teachings of Christianity, archaeologists would have no easy access to the symbolic meaning. Ideational cognitive archaeologists would establish this access by stipulating a connection to systems of meaning historically or ethnographically (e.g., through the Christian Bible). Archaeologists would have more direct access to the crucifix's iconic representation and perhaps also to its indexical reference. Much of prehistoric symbolic culture presents challenges as daunting as that of the crucifix.

Peirce provides a well-established theory of signs with which archaeologists can approach the archaeological record. It is necessary first to point out that archaeologists find the objects but must infer the interpretant and the sign. And, as in all archaeological arguments, the inferences must be appropriately warranted. The inferences must also respect parsimony. If a simpler version of interpretant can account for the object or pattern of objects, then it must be favored. To illustrate this approach, we turn to several well-known examples from the Palaeolithic.

(1) Hohlenstein-Stadel figurine (Fig. 1): This therianthrope is clearly iconic, but it is also universally acknowledged to be symbolic in a Peircean sense, and it is useful to dissect why. First, its status as a symbol is warranted by its familiarity. All modern people have experience with similar complex, multifaceted images as components of religious symbolism. The object in this case fits comfortably within a well-understood phenomenon. Moreover, such objects do not exist outside of such symbolic contexts, at least for modern people. It is this final caveat that should give us pause. Perhaps, life 40,000 years ago was different enough that, however unlikely it may seem, the object was not an arbitrary, conventional sign for anything. Additional evidence also warrants the symbolic attribution. Another ivory therianthrope, of similar age, has been found at the nearby site of Geissenklösterle (Conard, 2003), confirming the conventional *bona fides* of the artifact type. The object of the iconic reference is an imaginary creature made up of components of two different animals, components arbitrarily chosen and fused, which confirms the active role of symbolic reference in the conception of the artifact.

(2) Cave paintings: Upper Palaeolithic cave paintings (e.g., Fig. 11) are almost universally considered to be symbolic, but this conclusion is less sound than

the argument for the Hohlenstein-Stadel figurine. The paintings of animals are clearly iconic, but they are not necessarily symbolic in a Peircean sense; there is nothing conventional or arbitrary about them. The handprints are indexes but not necessarily symbols. It is only the geometric designs (Fig. 13)—chevrons, grids, dots, and lines—that warrant an inference of symbolism.

Given their location, they are not decorative, nor are they iconic. There is no apparent indexical linkage. We are left with two possibilities: (1) they are doodles done for the simple aesthetic pleasure of marking or (2) they are conventional, arbitrary signs (symbols) that stand for something else. The variety, sophistication, and location deep in caves associated with animal icons argues against the doodle explanation. Thus, parsimony favors symbolism.

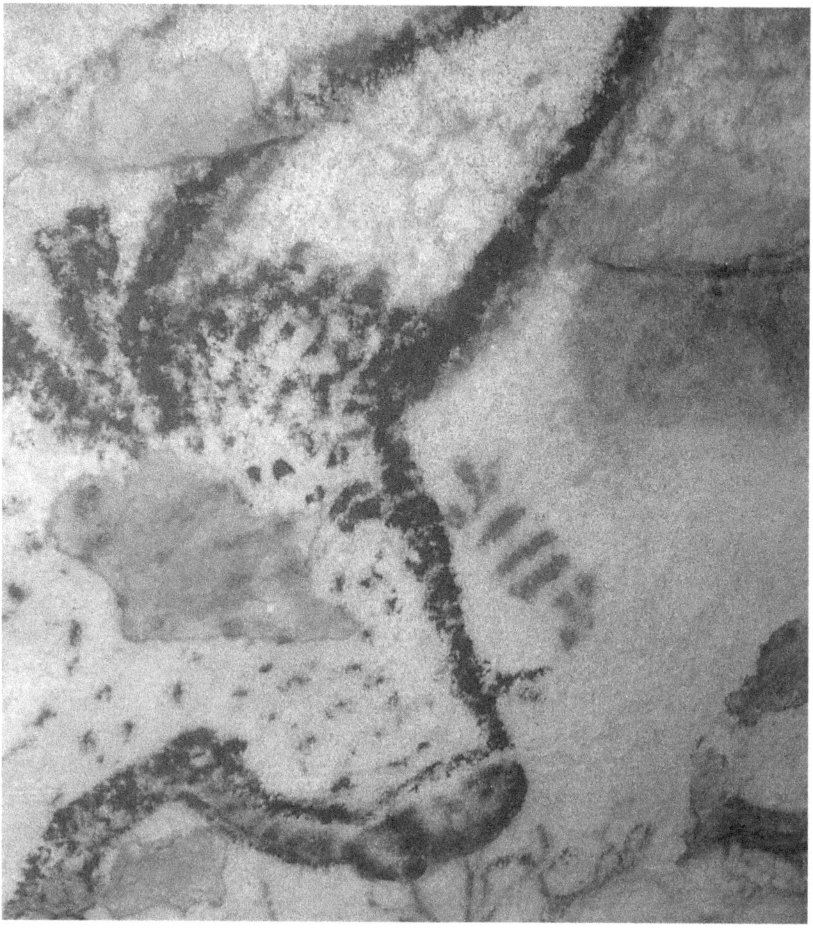

Figure 13 Polychrome geometric patterns from Lascaux, ca. 17–19,000. Wellcome Trust. CC BY 4.0.

(3) Mineral pigments: Most attributions of symbolism focus on nonutilitarian artifacts, which are artifacts that did not have a practical, mechanical role as tools. Hohlenstein-Stadel is a good example; the object could not have done any kind of practical work. Sometimes, however, evidence could be either utilitarian or nonutilitarian, and thus, it is necessary to add an inferential link that settles this ambiguity first. An example of this is the interpretation of mineral pigments. Ochres (varieties of iron oxide) and manganese oxides occur in archaeological sites dating back at least 300,000 years and have elicited claims for symbolic behavior. However, ethnographic and actualistic studies have demonstrated that mineral powders have a utilitarian function in hide processing and as binders in adhesives (Wadley et al., 2009). Thus, the simple presence of mineral pigments has two different sets of implications, only one of which suggests use as signs of some sort. Evidence from Twin Rivers, Zambia (Barham, 2002) (ca. 266–400,000) enabled Lawrence Barham to resolve this conundrum, at least for this site. Here, archaeologists excavated five different varieties (and colors) of ochre, obtained from different sources. Presumably, if an adhesive bonding agent was the goal, one variety would have been sufficient. The residents must have been interested in the different colors (Barham, 2002), most likely because they were coloring something. Because there were no tinted artifacts, the most likely target for the color was hominin bodies. The next link in the inference chain is the link to sign use. Was coloring bodies symbolic in a Peircean sense? Here, we must invoke parsimony. If one of the simpler varieties of object-sign interpretant could account for body coloring, it must be favored over arbitrary, conventional symbols. Iconicity is out; the pigments themselves do not resemble anything. Indexicality, on the other hand, is a real possibility. The colors might have acted as an extension of other things. Chris Knight (Knight, 2006; Knott, 2001) has the most memorable suggestion. He has suggested that the red ochres were stand-ins for menstrual blood; the color red was an extension (index) of menstrual fluids. In this way, women manipulated their identity in social interactions. Note that the reference is not conventional and arbitrary; it is thus not a true Peircean symbol. Of course, modern people continue to use pigments to manipulate identity (tattoos; makeup) and much of contemporary use is not narrowly symbolic, either. Here, the parsimonious decision goes against symbols and favors indexes.

(4) Neandertal symbolism: A few words about Neandertal symbolism are in order, given the saliency of Neandertals in popular science treatments of human evolution, and the unfortunate impression many archaeologists seem to have that this a primary interest of ECA. Over the past 20 years, evidence for Neandertal engagement with nonutilitarian material culture has accumulated (Zilhao et al., 2010), and all but the most dour skeptics accept it as reliable (Zilhao et al., 2010). There is now convincing evidence for shell and eagle talon pendants, use of eagle feathers, and mineral pigments.

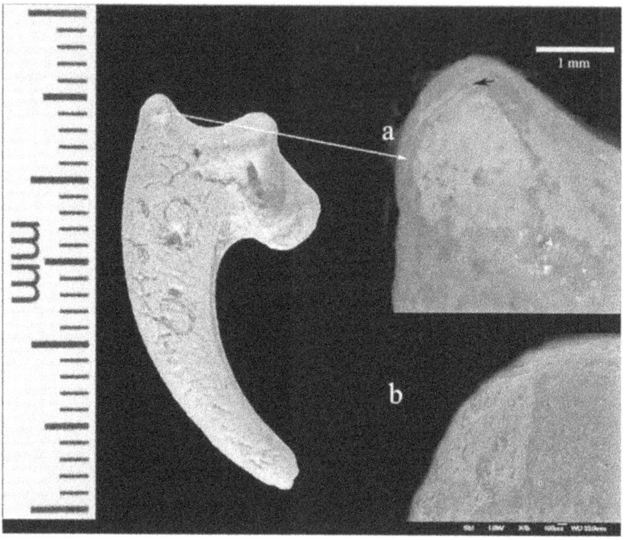

Figure 14 Neandertal pendant from Cueva Anton.

It is not abundant, but it supports attributing semiotic activities to our Neandertal cousins (see Botha, 2020 for detailed summary). But was it symbolic in a Peircean sense? As always, the cautious scholar (not typical for antagonists in this debate!) wields Occam's razor. After 150 years of Neandertal archaeology, no one has ever excavated or identified an iconic depiction of Neandertal origin, which is mildly puzzling if Neandertals were fully immersed in symbolic culture. However, there are modern humans who lack iconic depictions, or even forbid them altogether, so this lacuna is not too damning. Most of the Neandertal nonutilitarian material culture can be accounted for as aesthetic decorations or alterations of individual identity via use of ornaments and body coloring. As we have seen, the latter would be indexical usage, similar to the ochre use at Twin Rivers. Is it interesting to know this about Neandertal behavior? Certainly, it is. Must we conclude that Neandertal symbolism indicates that they were indistinguishable from modern humans (Wynn et al., 2016)? Certainly not. There are no reliably identified examples of Neandertal symbols in the Peircean sense. We would not be surprised if such evidence does come to light, but until then Neandertal semiotics and modern human semiotics should not be equated.

Semiotic ability is not a well-delineated cognitive ability. No one, at least to our knowledge, has made a controlled psychological study of the underpinnings of Peircean sign usage. We do not know how the cognitive requirements for icon use differ from the requirements for index use, or even if they do. There seems to be something more challenging about the use of arbitrary, conventional symbols, but only because there is neither a resemblance nor an extension that is easily available to perception. Despite this lack of cognitive clarity, evolutionary cognitive archaeologists must continue to engage the semiotic literature. Sign usage is an indispensable component of modern human life, and documenting its evolution is an important task for archaeologists. Cognitive archaeologists cannot treat it as an epiphenomenon. Formal theories of signs, such as Peirce's, remain the primary avenue for understanding.

Language

As challenging as interpretation of signs clearly is, language is harder. It is the Holy Grail for many who quest for the evolution of the human mind. It is arguably the most distinctive of human behaviors; it is so different from the communication systems of other animals that it is impossible to construct a continuum that encompasses them both. Some anthropologists have even averred that it is the defining feature of humanity. If science could provide an adequate account of the evolution of language, it would constitute a scholarly achievement on par with the documentation of human antiquity itself. Unfortunately, no such account is on the horizon, and it is unlikely that archaeology can do much to clarify the picture. Study of language evolution is one of the most contentious, and least productive, of the specialties in evolutionary science.

There are serious disagreements even at the level of basic definition; scholars cannot agree about what language is. Some linguists, such as Noam Chomsky, argue that language is enabled by a key grammatical ability to conceive of and execute a form of embedding known as recursion; if there is no recursion, there is no language (Hauser et al., 2002; Fitch et al., 2005). Others, such as Daniel Everett, argue that grammar is a minor component and that mastery of Peircean symbols is all that is required (Barham & Everett, 2020); once hominins achieved mastery of symbolic thinking, language must also have been present. Most linguists are more reluctant to use a single feature as definitional and instead use an extensive definition that includes symbols, grammar, rules of usage, and medium of delivery (e.g., speech) (Botha, 2020). Symbols and grammar have received most of the attention in discussions of evolution. For a communication system to qualify as linguistic, it must have both. Here, symbols have the Peircean or Saussurean meaning of standing for something via an arbitrary conventional link—in other words, words. Grammars are sets of rules for organizing words into longer utterances that have meanings that transcend the simple co-occurrence of the words ("man bites dog" is not the same as "dog bites man;" a word order rule changes the meaning).

Scholars approach the study of language evolution from an almost bewildering range of academic disciplines, not all of them scientific. These include animal behavior, zoology, comparative psychology, evolutionary psychology, developmental psychology, neuropsychology, structural linguistics, comparative linguistics, speech pathology, human genetics, paleontology, paleoanthropology, and archaeology. All provide modest insights, but none has provided a solution that persuades even a majority of scholars. Language evolution is a daunting topic of study because, until the advent of writing, literally nothing of language preserved in the evolutionary record. All arguments are by necessity indirect (Botha, 2020), requiring chains of inference. Indeed, Rudolf Botha developed his "windows approach," which we have borrowed from extensively in this book, to clarify the reasoning—and failures in reasoning—encountered in the vast literature on language evolution. Archaeologists fare slightly worse in Botha's critique than some other approaches, largely because of a laxity in definition and a tendency to avoid or skip lightly over necessary links in the chain of reasoning. However, archaeologists do study actual evidence of past behavior and thus have a role to play if they proceed with care. What can archaeologists hope to add?

As we discussed earlier in the chapter, archaeologists do have access to symbols; even if they cannot access the meaning of arbitrary symbols, they can often recognize that an artifact was a symbol or acted as platform for symbols. Archaeologists can therefore potentially provide chronological context for the symbolic component of language. There are challenges, of course, not the least of which is recognizing true arbitrary symbols, as opposed to context-rich indexes (driving a Ferrari is rife with indexical information, but it is not an arbitrary sign). Recently, Barham and Everett (2020) have taken an audacious stance that privileges archaeology as a means of documenting the evolution of language. They first define away much of the chaos surrounding language evolution: "language, defined here as communication based on symbols," (p. 2) with grammar playing a minor role, and "recursive grammar [Chomsky's essential component] a later and non-essential component of language." (p. 2). They then make explicit use of the Peircean classification of signs and suggest that the shared intention required for the manufacture of some handaxes implies not just indexicality but true symbolic signification. This places the advent of symbol use, and by extension language, at a very early date of >500,000 years. Most scholars interested in language evolution will probably balk at Barham and Everett's cavalier demotion of grammar's importance, but the stance may appeal to many archaeologists, who have had little success in documenting grammar in the archaeological record.

Grammars are sets of rules for stringing words together into utterances and sentences. Utterances and sentences are thus one-dimensional sequences of elements, typically words. Technical products also result from an ordered string of elements, typically actions. Perhaps, documentation of well-learned technical sequences could be evidence for grammatical thinking. This was the tack taken decades ago by Ralph Holloway (1969) and Glynn Isaac (1976) in two of the earliest examples of evolutionary cognitive archaeology. Though the stance seems sound initially, it runs afoul of a logical problem. Using technical rules as evidence for grammatical rules works only if the rule sets are the same kinds of things. If actors generate technical sequences using a different kind of rule generator, then the argument fails. In fact, people learn language and technical schemes very differently, and this obviates the relevance of technical sequences in a study of grammar. Children learn grammar effortlessly if they are raised in a linguistic milieu. No one ever learns even a simple technology effortlessly. Instead, technology requires observation, copying, failure, and repetition, often thousands of repetitions. This profound difference in learning suggests that technical routines and grammars have different neurological bases. One cannot be used as evidence for the other.

Stout et al. (Stout & Chaminade, 2007, 2012) have taken a slightly different approach to the dilemma. Instead of using technical sequences as evidence of grammar, they suggest that grammatical ability has evolutionary roots in technical cognition. Their approach is neuroarchaeological, which the reader will recall is based on neuroimaging and actualistic replication of prehistoric technology. They trained novice stone knappers over a two-year period and imaged their brains at set intervals using fMRI, which measures blood flow, diffusion tensor imaging, and fractional anisotropy (which trace white matter tracts). They found that learning these motor skills produces significant changes in the brain, including frontoparietal areas of the brain that support language (Hecht et al., 2014). On the basis of this neurological evidence, they suggest that toolmaking and language coevolved in human evolution. This is an important and provocative conclusion that, if corroborated, would be the most significant archaeological contribution to date to the understanding of language evolution. It does not reveal anything about grammar per se, but it does raise the possibility that initial grammatical regularities drew on patterns of motor organization.

Section III

Brief Outline of Hominin Cognitive Evolution

Summaries of human evolution typically take a narrative approach organized chronologically, beginning with the first recognized hominins some 5 million years ago and closing with the end of the Pleistocene geologic epoch about 12,000 years ago, at which point human hunter-gatherers occupied most of the planet. Such narratives summarize fossil, archaeological, environmental, and geographic evidence and present a story of continuous development in which we humans are the protagonists. Embedded in the accounts are unspecified theoretical assumptions, unsupported bridges spanning immense gaps in evidence and time, and unacknowledged biases. There are, as the adage notes, serious devils in the details. Nevertheless, we are going to attempt such a narrative in order to demonstrate the potential of evolutionary cognitive archaeology to inform us about the evolution of the human mind. We will not attempt a comprehensive narrative; we will shamelessly pass over controversies about fossils and genetics and population histories. Instead, we will focus narrowly on the archaeological evidence for hominin cognition organized chronologically into three divisions that we think encompass major phases of hominin cognitive development. We will also throw in a bit about Neanderthals because they have become popular doppelgängers for modern humans.

DOI: 10.4324/9781003014485-14

12 Phase 1

The Bipedal Apes—3.3–1.7 Million

The first hominins diverged from the other African apes sometime before 7 million years ago (Ma). The evolutionary divergence coincided with significant shifts in African environments, especially a shrinkage of continuous canopy tropical forests and expansion of woodlands and grasslands. Anatomically, the divergence included a dramatic shift in locomotion to bipedalism and a dietary shift that selected for thick enamel on the molars and a reduction in canine size. Initially, there was no significant shift away from African ape-sized brains, and thus for several million years, this new branch of African apes adapted to a locomotor/dietary niche that did not select for any dramatically new cognitive abilities. But, as anthropoids closely related to chimpanzees, some, perhaps all, of these early hominins were tool users.

Several modern anthropoids, including New World monkeys (*Cebus* sp.), Old World monkeys (*Macaca* sp.), and apes, use tools, which suggests that tool use evolved independently on several occasions, and each time, it arose via the object manipulation propensity of anthropoid hands and the neural network that supports it (Orban & Caruana, 2014; Orban et al., 2006). Although it is perhaps misleading to generalize, most anthropoid tool use involves access to embedded or guarded foods. Cebus monkeys use stone hammers to break open nuts, and macaques use stones to crack open mollusks, but the most extensive tool-based foraging belongs to hominins' closest relatives, the chimpanzees. In West Africa, chimpanzee communities use stones to crack open hard-shelled nuts and in the process generate a great deal of waste. In East Africa, chimpanzee communities use probes to extract termites from their mounds and ants from their nests. Indeed, such extractive foraging with tools is common enough to qualify as a significant component of the chimpanzee niche. It also produces an archaeological record that "primate archaeologists" have begun to exploit as another method of primate ethology (Whiten et al., 2009). Early hominins did not evolve from chimpanzees, but given their phylogenetic propinquity, they are the best model for the tool-using component of very early hominin niches. When interpreting the archaeological evidence of the first stone tools, it is more appropriate first to compare them to this chimpanzee model than to invoke a human model. Early hominins were, after all, bipedal apes.

DOI: 10.4324/9781003014485-15

The oldest stone tools yet identified, and the *de facto* advent of the archaeological record, date to 3.3 Ma from Lomekwi 3 in Kenya (Harmand et al., 2015). The hominin responsible was probably a variety of East African *Australopithecus*. The second oldest stone tools are 2.6 Ma from Gona in Ethiopia, a mere 700,000 years later (Semaw, 2000). This is a long time, and there is a very real possibility that hominins of various types developed a knapped lithic technology numerous times but lost it almost as many times. If it was initially a minor component of the niche and if its continuance depended on a challenging form of observational learning, then loss was predictable. It was not until close to 2 Ma that a system of knapping appears to have "caught on" to become both important to the niche and reliably transferable from one generation to the next. This knapping system was a component of a meat eating/butchery adaptation, probably tied to scavenging. In many respects, it remained very ape-like, but there are indications that cognitive changes away from an ape-like solution had begun to accrue.

Nick Toth and Kathy Schick (Toth & Schick, 2018), in an excellent summary of this early evidence, list 17 African localities that date to before 1.7 Ma, most of them in Ethiopia, Kenya, and Tanzania where they are associated with deposits in the East African Rift Valley system. By standards of more recent time periods, these "Oldowan" sites were small, ranging from 3 to 400 m^2. They consisted of thin scatters of stone tools, knapping debris, and in some cases comminuted bone. Most of sites were close to water, typically in deltaic deposits or lake edges, and most were situated within a few hundred meters of the gravel deposits from which the knappers acquired their raw material. Because

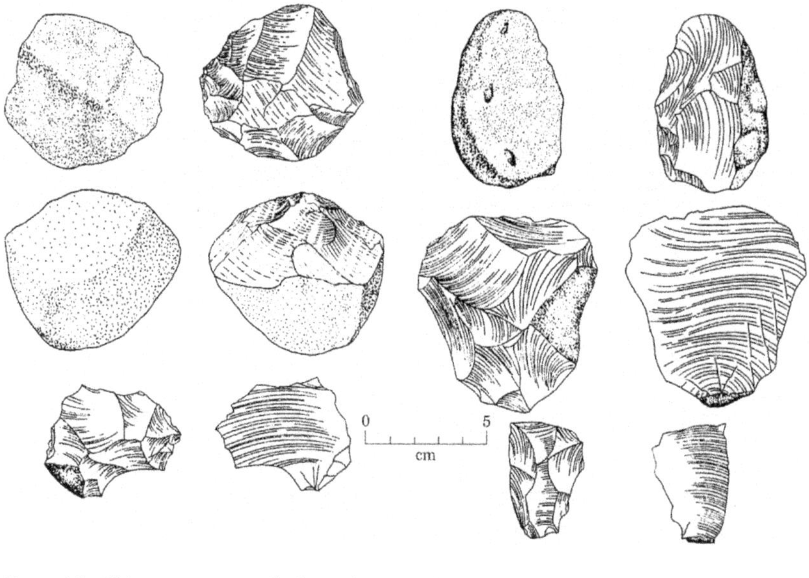

Figure 15 Oldowan stone tools from the site of Gona, 2.6 Ma. After Semaw, 2000.

the archaeological remains consist of little other than lithics, archaeologists have focused a good deal of attention on reconstructing knapping procedures. The most informative methods have been actualistic replication and core refitting to document *chaînes opératoires* (Delagnes & Roche, 2005; Stout et al., 2009; Toth, 1987). The Oldowan knappers used two forms of knapping: free-hand direct percussion, in which the knapper held a "core" in one hand and struck it with a stone "hammer" held in the other, and "bipolar" technique, in which the knapper held a core on a solid substrate (e.g., a patch of bedrock or a stone anvil) and struck it with a stone hammer. The hominins selected the best available raw material, lava and quartzite cobbles being optimal for this kind of knapping. They typically acquired these cobbles from nearby gravel deposits, but at a few of the sites hominins carried cobbles of high-quality stone over 10 km (Braun et al., 2009). Because little other than stone has survived, the uses to which these tools were put are poorly known. The presence of fractured bones with cutmarks clearly establishes butchery, and pitted stones suggest pounding, perhaps nuts or underground storage organs of plants (Mora & de la Torre, 2005). Both must have been components of the niche, but there was also likely to have been archaeologically invisible varieties of tool use. What does this meagre record suggest about cognitive abilities?

Not surprisingly, most of what archaeologists can reconstruct concerns the making and use of stone tools. Actualistic replication and use, and *chaînes opératoires* from refitted cores suggest that this first phase of hominin cognitive evolution witnessed agonizingly slow, almost imperceptible developments in cognition.

Memory

There is little indication that the long-term memory capacity of these early hominins differed significantly from that of living apes. The amount of stored information required to make and use stone tools did not clearly exceed the stored information required for chimpanzee tool use, but this is of course very difficult to measure, even with living subjects. Most of the information consisted of motor procedures. There were no normative types. Instead, the range of products reflected the range of procedures. The hominins must have had explicit, nonsemantic, long-term memories—for example, "lava flakes well," "sandstone does not"—all nonsemantic. There are glimmers of working memory in action. Cognitive control, an important component of the central executive, is evident in refitted cores from Lokalalei 2C and from some of the reconstructed sequences from Gona (Delagnes & Roche, 2005; Semaw et al., 2009) The refitted cores record episodes of core rejuvenation. These were knapping blows directed at maintaining core productivity rather producing large useful flakes. This is a simple example of task switching, which is a cognitive control function. But again, despite the seeming complexity, it does not exceed the task switching demonstrated by chimpanzees probing for termites, who maintain the stiffness of the probe and monitor tunnel entrances.

What core rejuvenation does establish is that stone knapping relied on both working memory and long-term memory, which is true of modern expert technical systems. It is thus possible to trace the evolution of stone knapping as the evolution of expert cognition.

Spatial Cognition

The hard hammer percussion routines provide evidence for developments in visuospatial attention. In Toth's experiments teaching the bonobo Kanzi to knap stone, Kanzi never learned to examine cores for usable striking platforms. He either bashed the hammer and core together or threw the hammer at the core (his preferred technique) (Toth et al., 1993, 2006). Even the earliest examples of hominin knapping included identification of potential platforms. This required close visual searching and an ability to discriminate knappable platforms in the visuospatial field of the core. While this is not spatial cognition *per se*, it is a component of the visuospatial sketchpad of working memory. Beyond this, the spatial cognition of the early hominins resembled that of apes, that is, arranging action in space using topological relationships such as inside/outside, a boundary dividing a spatial field, and ordered placement of elements (Wynn, 1989, 2002). At the larger scale of landscape use, the sources of raw material indicate that the hominins habitually carried cobbles and chunks of raw material hundreds of meters and often several kilometers. This arguably placed a load on spatial memory, but again it need not have significantly exceeded that of chimpanzees, who have excellent memories for locations of fruit trees.

Technical Cognition

Actualistic replication of Oldowan artifacts, core refitting, most notably from Lokalalei 2C (Delagnes & Roche, 2005; Roche & Texier, 1995), and tracing the movement of artifacts across the landscape have been the basis of claims for cognitive "complexity" beyond anything known for living apes (Hovers, 2012; Toth & Schick, 2018). Few of these technical analyses have been grounded in cognitive theory, and thus, there is little basis for assessing these claims. However, they have identified action patterns that appear to require higher levels of manual skill (hand-eye coordination) than what is known for apes. There were also sets of interrelated actions that had more components, and more dependent actions, than anything known from ape technology. In this sense, the Oldowan was technically more complex. We mentioned earlier that the Oldowan knappers monitored cores as they knapped, a working memory task. They also demonstrated persistence in reducing cores to the point at which the cores could no longer yield useful flakes, and this task persistence, unlinked to immediate need, is unknown for apes (e.g., chimpanzees do not continue making probes after acquiring one workable example). The hominins were able to recognize different raw materials and invariably selected the raw material that yielded sharp, durable flakes. They also carried raw material from source to site of use and occasionally carried flakes on to yet another locale (Toth & Schick, 2018). Sometimes they tested raw material at the source; telltale cortical flakes are often missing from sites of use. Other times, they carried in untested cobbles and tested them at the site of use (evidence of single flake removals, or crush marks from testing blows). The tools were primarily butchery tools. The sharp flakes were effective slicing tools, and the cobbles and cores were good for bashing into bones for marrow. Yes, this technical system had more going on than, say, chimpanzees using hammers to forage for nuts, but without a theoretical context, it is not clear that it represents *cognitive* complexity.

Miriam Haidle and colleagues (Lombard et al., 2019) have taken a more systematic approach using her cognigrams, which are a form of *chaînes opératoires* focused on hominin shifts in attention and problem-solution distance, a measure of the steps separating initiation of action and completion. Their 2019 article directly compared capuchin monkeys using rock pounding to crack open nuts, chimpanzees using hammer and anvil to open coula nuts, and the knapping procedure evident at Lomekwi 3, the oldest knapping evidence yet found at 3.3 million. The comparison is thorough and systematic. Moreover, by inferring attention and problem-solution distance, the authors infer cognitively relevant components of the procedures. They conclude that "it would appear that the Lomekwian knappers were able to handle longer problem-solution distances compared to pounding capuchin monkeys and nut-cracking chimpanzees" (p. 72). They also invoke the cognitive model of expert cognition and retrieval structures (see the following section), which emphasizes an interacting system of long-term memory and working memory and suggest that the Lomekwi knapping required enhancements in memory chunking and chaining.

Social Cognition

The dearth of very early sites, their small size, and the apparent ephemeral nature of their occupation means that social cognition is largely inaccessible to direct archaeological enquiry. Most interpretations of early hominin social life rely on analogy to nonhuman primate social behavior. The one exception to this poverty is social learning. Over the last decade, a lively debate has arisen about how early hominins learned to knap (Gärdenfors & Högberg, 2017; Morgan et al., 2015; Putt et al., 2014; Tennie et al., 2017).

On the one side of the debate stand Gärdenfors and Högberg (2017), who argue that the complex motor sequences of stone knapping could not be learned by observation and practice and that some kind of instruction had to have occurred. "We conclude that transmitting Oldowan technology requires imitation, including rehearsal, together with active teaching in the form of evaluative feedback, drawing attention, and most importantly, demonstration" (p. 197). Moreover, demonstration required "advanced mind reading" for both the teacher and the learner (the teacher knows that the learner does not know, and the learner knows that the teacher knows something useful). Tennie et al. (2017), on the other hand, argue that early knapping could have been largely a matter individual learning, with perhaps some "low-fidelity" social learning. One way out of the impasse is via experimentation and actualistic studies. Morgan et al. (2015), for example, used a serial learning paradigm in which sets of novices learned to knap using different forms of social learning, including no social learning (participants were simply provided with artifacts and raw material), imitation, and active teaching. They in turn became the models/teachers for a second set of novices learning from them in the same way. Knappers who learned by active teaching were better able to pass along the appropriate knowledge than those who learned by imitation or individual learning. The archaeological record also has important evidence to add to the mix. In Delagne's and Roche's (2005) influential account of refitting cores from Lokalalei 2C, the knappers all appear to have followed the same basic procedure, which implies that some form of high-fidelity social learning was in play (Gärdenfors & Högberg, 2017; Morgan et al., 2015; Putt et al., 2014; Tennie et al., 2017; Wynn & Coolidge, 2016). Stout et al. came to a similar conclusion about the earlier sites at Gona (Pargeter et al., 2019), but support the insight using statistical analyses of flaking products and experimental replication. They conclude that individual learning could not have produced the uniform knapping strategy evident from the Gona sites and that some form of high fidelity-copying was necessary. They do not, however, suggest that teaching was necessary.

The consensus would appear to be that the kinds of hard hammer knapping evident at even the earliest sites required some form of high-fidelity copying in which novices observed and reproduced motor procedures. Even if active demonstration was not required, this still suggests a more intimate and continuous interaction between novices and experts than one ever sees for nonhuman primates. This in turn suggests the use of shared attention, which is a low-level ToM.

Symbolism, Language, and Aesthetics

There is nothing in the first 1.6 million years of the archaeological record that speaks directly, one way or the other, about language. All the arguments about language for this early time period rely on fossil evidence, primate evidence, or features of language itself. There is also almost no archaeological evidence for symbols or aesthetics. But there is the Makapansgat Pebble.

This is a pebble of jasperite, about 8 cm in diameter, with a naturally occurring primate-like face. A local schoolteacher found the artifact on the surface at the 2.5 Ma eponymous *Australopithecus* site and gave it to Raymond Dart, who excavated the site. Jasperite is not a local rock type; someone carried the pebble to Makapansgat. The provenience is obviously a challenge, but there is no reason to think a modern human was the agent. If the agent was an *Australopithecus*, must we conclude that the artifact was symbolic? It clearly is iconic. Archaeologists of the deep past must wield Occam's razor often, but with care. The artifact was almost certainly not a symbol in the Peircean sense of carrying

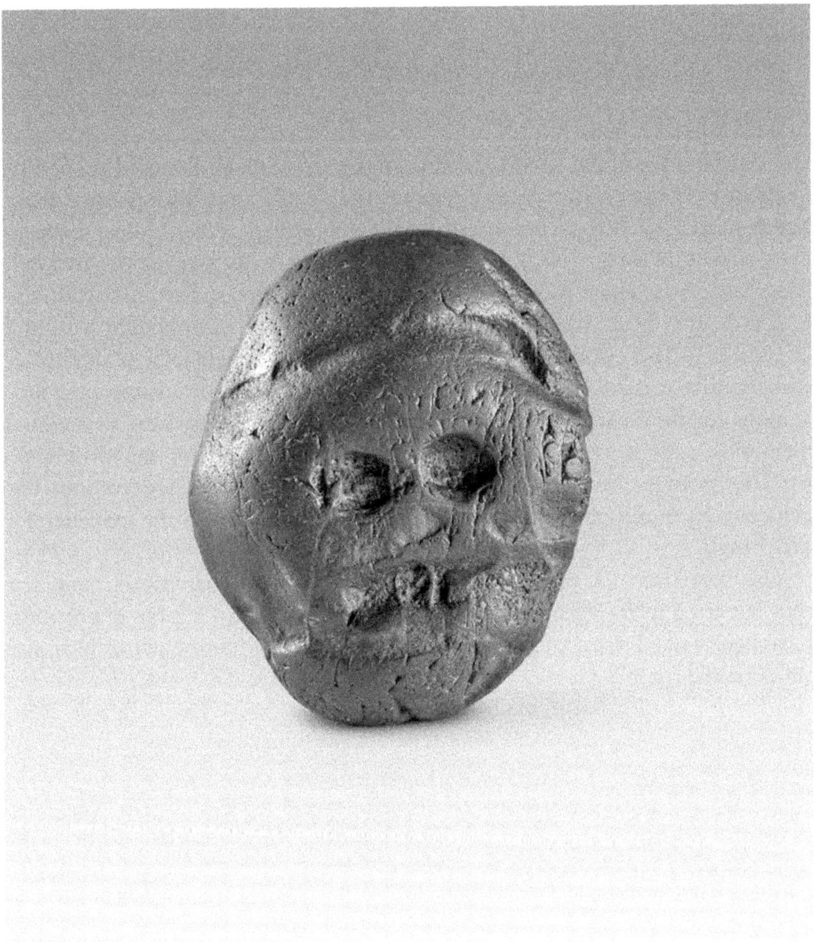

Figure 16 Makapansgat pebble with pareidolic face, 2.5 Ma, 8 cm. After Berlant & Wynn, 2018.

arbitrary reference. Anthropoid primates are very good at detecting faces; it is an important component of social interaction. If an *Australopithecus* examined the pebble, it would have recognized the face immediately. No symbolic thinking was necessary. This leaves two questions: why examine the pebble and why carry it away? The first is easy. Stone knappers examine stones, especially a stone of this size and raw material; it might make a useful core or hammerstone. But why carry it somewhere? It does not have the crushing typical of a hammerstone and was never flaked. Perhaps, the carrier simply lost it. Or, perhaps, the face gave the finder pleasure, amusement, or wonder. We clearly will never know, but eventually hominins did invest artifacts with pleasing shapes, a development that may have been preceded by collecting pleasing objects (Berlant & Wynn, 2018).

Summary

Our examination of this very early phase of the archaeological record has identified relatively few cognitive developments that would have distinguished these bipeds from their African ape cousins. The archaeological record is so sparse as to be almost invisible—a handful of sites for a span of over one-and-a-half million years. Yet, it seems probable that knapping and using stone tools over these long millennia could well have changed the way these apes thought with and about tools. The evidence has provided hints. Core management implicates the cognitive control functions of working memory. The various knapping procedures required expert retrieval structures with more long-term procedural memories, more sustained visual attention, and more working memory capacity. The knappers learned via shared attention and high-fidelity copying. The evidence for scavenging and butchery is commensurate with the evidence for knapping.

This very short list probably cannot account for the increase in brain size that occurred in the *Homo* line about 2.4 Ma. Selection for large brains must have been linked to behaviors archaeologists either cannot detect or have not yet detected.

13 Phase 2

The Axe Age—
1.7 Million–300,000 Years Ago

Between 1.8 million years ago and 300,000 years ago, hominin cognition evolved from ape-like to human-like. Hominins, probably an early variety of *Homo erectus*, began leaving Africa before 1.8 Ma and soon occupied most of the warmer regions of Asia and Europe. The appellation bipedal ape no longer applied; there was little ape-like about *Homo erectus*. The list of evolutionary firsts associated with *Homo erectus* is quite long, including: first hominin with a modern body size; first with modern sexual dimorphism; first to leave Africa; adapt to life on grasslands; live at higher altitudes (>2,000 m); hunt large animals; and sleep on the ground. By 300,000 years ago (300 Ka), hominins, now varieties of *Homo heidelbergensis*, had added many more, including a brain size that was in the modern range, adaptations to higher latitudes, and control of fire. This phase encompassed many of the most significant developments in hominin behavioral evolution. Unfortunately, we cannot document these developments in much detail; the archaeological record remains spotty, spanning as it does 1.5 million years and three continents. There were also several successive varieties of hominin, not all of whom were ancestors of ours. These, too, left archaeological traces. By 300 Ka, they had diversified and adapted to local conditions, making generalizations precarious. High-quality archaeological sites with excellent preservation are few, but museum drawers contain millions of stone tools. Used judiciously, they have a fascinating story to tell. We begin with technical cognition because it left the most reliable signature.

Technical Cognition

The most salient and enigmatic development in lithic technology was the handaxe.

To date, the best definition of the handaxe is a description penned by John Gowlett (2006) that emphasizes the ergonomic features of this tool. The label "handaxe" is a little misleading; they were hand-held tools but were rarely, if ever, used as axes. They are large core tools, typically over 10 cm in length and often much larger. The thickness and breadth concentrate mass toward one end, which Gowlett termed a "glob-butt." Ergonomically, this is the center of gravity and optimal place to grip the tool. Handaxes were hand-held cutting

DOI: 10.4324/9781003014485-16

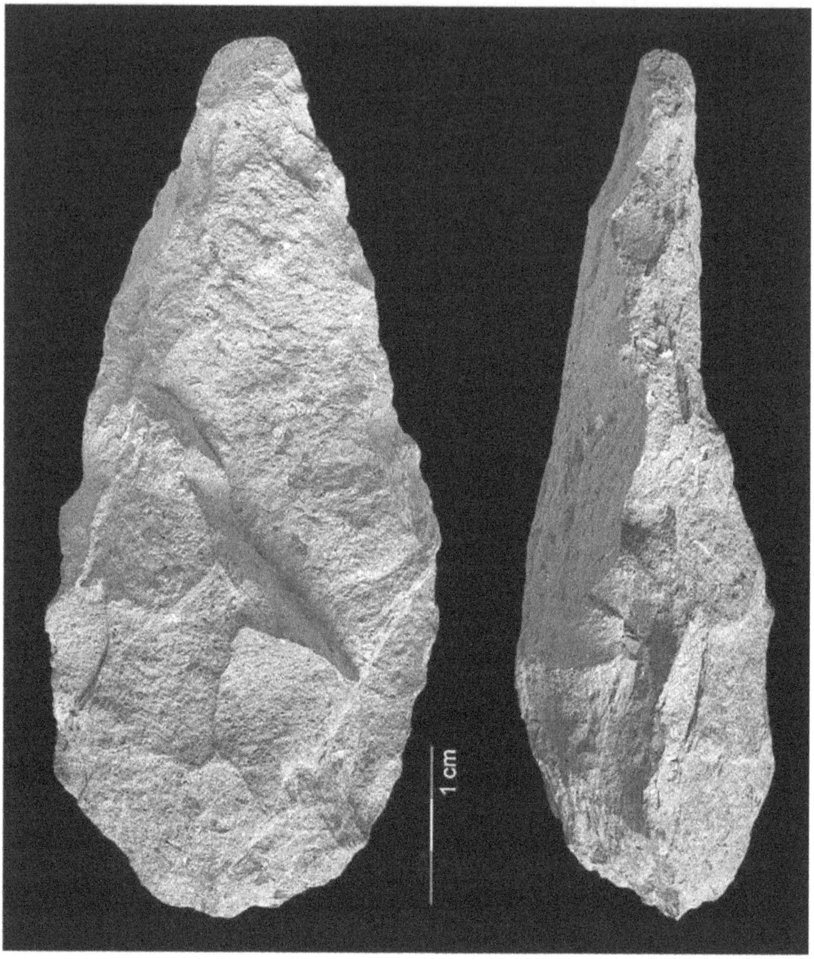

Figure 17 Giant handaxe from FLK West, 1.69 Ma (Diez-Martin et al., 2019).

tools, and "forward extension" maximizes length of cutting edge. Handaxes have bifacially trimmed edges around most of the perimeter; this "edge maintenance" produces a sturdy, durable cutting edge. Long, narrow hand tools tend to twist in use. Handaxe makers reduced this tendency by incorporating "lateral extension" perpendicular to the length; this also produced a characteristic teardrop shape. Weight is literally tiring, and the knappers reduced weight by thinning the artifact ("thickness control"). Finally, the hominins often imposed a "skewness" to the shape to optimize grip and cutting edge orientation. Thus, handaxes were clusters of ergonomic features. These features had coalesced into a single artifact over hundreds of millennia as hominins relied more and more on large core tools for heavy work. But there was a bit more to them; the knappers paid attention to overall shape.

Consider the very large handaxe in Fig. 17. Diez-Martin et al. (2019) have analyzed the knapping sequence used to make this 1.69 Ma artifact, and it is clear that the knapper intended to impose a bilateral symmetry (more later on the symmetry). This did not enhance the ergonomic potential of the artifact in any way, so why did he or she invest the extra effort to do this? The exact "why" may be out of reach, but something quite important is evident—the knapper was thinking *about* the artifact. This seemingly simple development marked a watershed in the relationship between hominins and their tools. Tools were now a category of object, ontologically distinct from the procedures to accomplish a task. We suspect this shift occurred through curation. As hominins invested more effort in making large core tools, it paid to carry them after use rather than abandon them. This extended their presence in attention into the future and the past and slowly transformed the ergonomic cluster into a tool concept (Gilbert, 2018; Malafouris, 2021; Overmann, 2021; Wynn, 2021). And once the handaxe was a permanent feature of daily existence, this "thinking about" opened up other possible roles.

Diez-Martin's analysis also documents cognitive control components of working memory. In an fMRI study of handaxe manufacture, Stout et al. (2015) identified neural localities activated during visualization of handaxe production that did not appear during visualization of Oldowan-like knapping. One of these localities, the *pars triangularis* of the inferior right frontal lobe, is generally associated with cognitive control. The description of the flaking sequence for the FLK W giant handaxe suggests that the knapper tracked three goals while making the artifact: (1) thinning the large heavy tool (Gowlett's thickness control), (2) production of two converging bifacial edges (forward extension and edge maintenance), and (3) mirroring one lateral edge with the other. He or she flipped the artifact over several times and modified the overall form using discontinuous flaking sequences. This required the interruption of the rhythmic knapping action, recommencing at another location. This is a cognitive control challenge, implicating response inhibition and task switching specifically (Diez-Martin et al., 2019).

Evidence from the Israeli site of Gesher Benot Ya'aqov (GBY—ca. 780,000 Ka) corroborates Diez-Martin's analysis and adds important additional pieces to the puzzle of handaxe technical cognition (Herzlinger et al., 2017). Here, the hominins used several different and distinct technical procedures for producing the large flake blanks that were the first step in the production of handaxes and cleavers (a core tool similar to a handaxe, but with a "bit" at the end instead of a tip). The knappers decided at the time they quarried the stone which variety of tool to make and which procedure to follow. They carried the blanks away to be completed at GBY. Thus, their technical procedures were embedded in their system of landscape use. The procedures also had a nested structure of routines and subroutines. Herzlinger et al. suggest that GBY technical cognition was expert cognition, engaging long-term memory and working memory via retrieval structures, and was thus similar in overall organization to modern craft production, though with lower demands on long-term memory. Herzlinger et al. also make the more provocative suggestion that the alternative procedures were distinct enough to have warranted semantic labels.

The GBY hominins also used expert cognition when processing animals and plants. The exceptional preservation at GBY includes the remains of 55 species of edible plants, including prickly water lilies, whose use required "scheduling according to life-cycle of the plant, diving to recover nuts, carrying with containers of some sort, drying and cleaning, roasting, and pounding to pop or remove the shells. . . .The activity required two dependent but temporally disjunct phases" (Alperson-Afil et al., 2020), separated by hours, even days. Such a procedure requires prospective memory, in addition to the long-term and working memory components evident in other GBY procedures.

The evidence for controlled fire at GBY is the oldest widely accepted evidence in the archaeological record. Fire maintenance itself requires a sophisticated technical procedure (Twomey, 2013), which is commensurate with the other evidence at GBY. There are earlier possible examples of fire use stretching all the way back to 1.4 Ma (Chazan, 2017; Walker et al., 2016; Wrangham, 2009), and it is possible, even likely, that fire use was a component of Phase 2 niches since the beginning. The difficulty is that direct remains of ash and charcoal do not survive beyond about 300,000 years, and archaeologists must rely on less direct traces such as heat modified bone or stone. Given that these hominins no longer slept in trees, fire use would have been a boon to security. Wrangham also argues persuasively that cooking was not only possible, but necessary for digesting meat (Wrangham, 2009).

In most respects, the technical cognition of these early *Homos* was more human-like than ape-like. However, there was also something that was archaic and unimaginative. Technical change was virtually absent. The GBY stratigraphic sequence spans a period of about 50,000 years, and over that time, there was not a single new technology added. Over the entire 1.5-million-year span of the Axe Age, there were only a handful of innovations in lithic technology, mostly tied to core management. This suggests that conscious invention of new technologies never occurred and that innovations accumulated via errors and other serendipitous processes (Wynn & Coolidge, 2014). The absence of invention suggests in turn that these hominins lacked the folk physics of causality that is a component of mechanical reasoning in modern human technology.

Spatial Cognition

The rare technical developments that did accrue between 1.8 Ma and 300,000 Ka document evolution in hominin spatial cognition. The earliest of these was the coordination of the two primary visual processing streams (Wynn, 2002, 2010): the dorsal stream that processes spatial relations and the ventral stream that processes shape recognition. Knapping is primarily a spatial guided motor procedure (Stout et al., 2000) that relies on the dorsal pathway. Recognizing and creating symmetry relies on ventral processing. The knappers of the FLK West giant handaxe needed to coordinate these two processing streams. Nonhuman primates do not impose shape on tools nor did Oldowan hominins. The brain region that does this for modern humans is in the superior temporal sulcus (Liu et al., 2019). The ability to detect symmetry is an old evolutionary development linked to predator and food detection, but the motivation to impose symmetry seems limited to hominins.

1.7-million-year-old hominins also produced spheroids—stone balls—and these are a bigger puzzle. Unlike handaxes, whose ergonomics are fairly clear, the spheroids do not have a clear known function. They might have been projectiles, as Louis Leakey suggested 90 years ago (Leakey, 1931), but then they would not have needed to be round, or they might have been bashing tools (Toth & Schick, 1986), but this, too, would not dictate such spherical forms. We suspect, once again, that hominins took pleasure in producing these forms.

The second major development in spatial cognition, allocentric perception, occurred much later, after 800 Ka, and perhaps not fully engaged until 500 Ka. Allocentric perception is the ability to imagine an alternative viewpoint not centered on ego. This is an especially useful ability for navigation because it enables a traveler to recognize familiar landmarks seen from a new angle. Evolutionary psychologist Irwin Silverman (Silverman et al., 2007) has argued that it evolved in support of hunting. It would certainly have been a useful ability for hominins exploiting large territories or pioneering in new habitats. The evidence for allocentric perception comes, yet again, from handaxes. Late handaxes, after 800,000, have three-dimensional symmetry—plan, profile, and cross-section. The third, cross-section, is not available to direct perception; it must be imagined. This required allocentric perception.

Sleep quality may have facilitated the evolution of spatial cognition. With the advent of *Homo erectus*, hominins abandoned sleeping in nests in trees. They had a larger body size than earlier hominins, which reduced the number of useable trees, but more importantly, they had moved out into more open habitats with much smaller trees. Sleeping on the ground would have allowed longer, more coherent sleep episodes (Coolidge & Wynn, 2006; Coolidge, 1974), and expansion of REM sleep. Quality sleep facilitates memory consolidation, especially for procedural and spatial information (Coolidge & Wynn, 2006). Perhaps, it was not entirely coincidence that enhanced technical and spatial cognition coincided with the advent of ground sleep. Of course, there were also downsides; even large hominins sleeping on the ground face increased predation. This danger could have been mitigated by staggered sleep schedules (owls vs. larks), fire maintenance, or larger groups.

The spatial cognition of hominins was essentially modern by 500,000 years ago. In a sense, our ability to locate ourselves in space and navigate novel routes is an old ability. We have recently enhanced our spatial abilities with tools, but the core neurological resources have been placed since the time of *Homo heidelbergensis*.

Aesthetic Cognition

Art may be a recent, modern human acquisition, but aesthetic thinking is much older. Earlier, we discussed how the Makapansgat pebble with the emoji face might have reflected an aesthetic appreciation, but it was not a modified object. Phase 1 hominins did not aestheticize their tools. Phase 2 hominins did.

No surprise, handaxes were the vehicle. In our earlier discussion of handaxe symmetry, we did not speculate about why hominins might have imposed symmetry on artifacts, but Derek Hodgson has (Hodgson, 2000, 2006). When the visual system detects certain salient patterns, it sends signals to the pleasure centers of the brain. Thus, making a symmetry was a pleasurable activity. The visual system also responds to other kinds of "implicit visual effects," as cognitive psychologist Helmut Leder terms them (Leder et al., 2004; Leder & Nadal, 2014). If a pattern elicits pleasure, an exaggeration elicits greater pleasure. This is the peak shift effect, and it played a role in handaxe production through size (gigantism) and fineness of finish (Fig. 18, Kathu Pan) (Berlant & Wynn, 2018). Hominin knappers also selected attractive stone, even if it was more difficult to work. By half-a-million years ago, they were producing some stunning results.

But to what end? Gregory Currie (Currie & Zhu, 2021) suggests that the simple visual pleasure scenario is "too thin" an account of the handaxe aesthetic and embraces a "hand of the maker" scenario in which knappers used handaxes on occasion to advertise their skill. Interestingly, artist Tony Berlant favors this stance as well, based on his experience assessing distinctive "hands" of contemporary artists, Navajo weavers, and Mimbres ceramics. For Berlant, the exceptional handaxes document an urge to create, an aesthetic impulse, more than just a need to advertise (Berlant & Wynn, 2018). The handaxes were the canvas on which this aesthetic impulse played out.

Social Cognition

Primate intelligence and cognition appear to be socially driven to a large degree. In the 1980s, primatologists Richard Byrne and Andrew Whiten proposed the Machiavellian hypothesis, which emphasized primates' use of tactical deception (Byrne & Whiten, 1988), and in the 1990s and 2000s, evolutionary psychologist Robin Dunbar developed the Social Brain Hypothesis (Dunbar, 1998; Dunbar et al., 2010), which emphasizes affiliative behaviors such as grooming that enhance group cohesion. Life in permanent social groups that included adult males is the challenge that primates have had to solve, according to these hypotheses, and it has selected for a variety of cognitive abilities, including sophisticated abilities to read and anticipate the action of others. Dunbar (1993) documented a provocative correlation between the size of primate's neocortex and the average size of its social group. Thus, *a priori*, any discussion of the evolution of hominin cognition must consider the likelihood that social cognition may have been the primary selective agent.

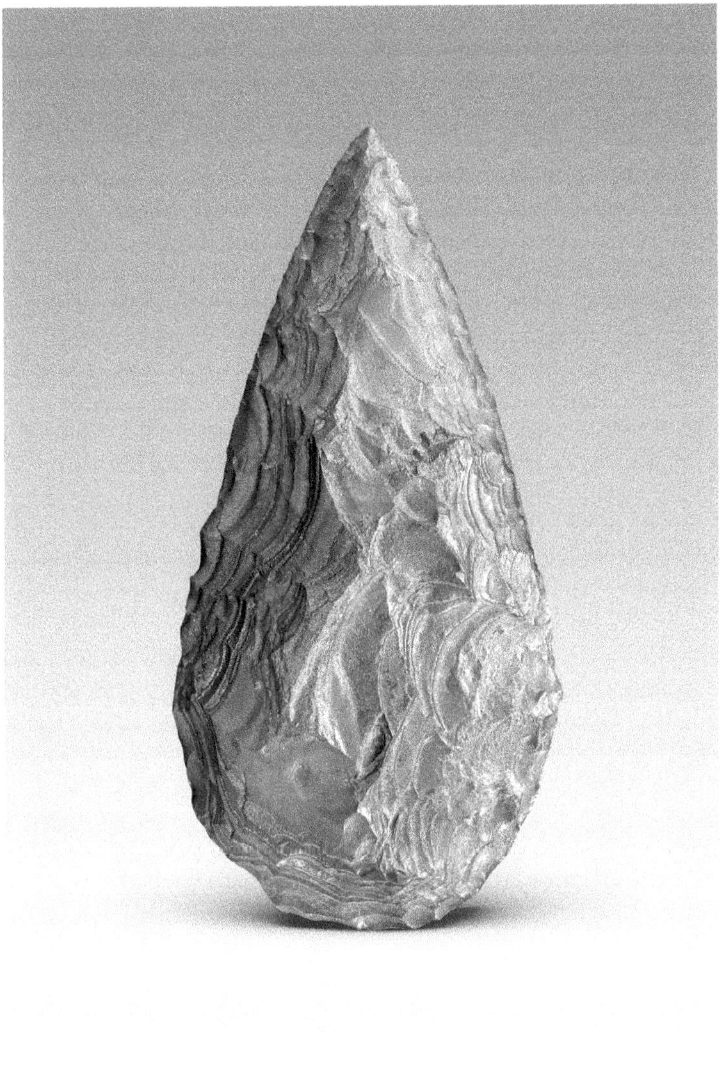

Figure 18 Kathu Pan, South Africa, 23.4 × 10.8 cm, ca. 500,000. After Berlant & Wynn, 2018. With permission of Nasher Sculpture Center.

Significant social changes accompanied the advent of *Homo erectus*. Foremost was a reduction in sexual dimorphism; females were now much closer to males in size. For primates, this typically signals a reduction in intermale aggression. Also, larger size placed increased caloric demands on pregnant and lactating females. Combined with the altriciality required by larger brained neonates, this suggests some kind of assistance, either from males (most likely) or from mothers' mothers (less likely if, like other African apes, *Homo erectus* was male philopatric). The new social dynamics put selection pressure on social cognition. Social behavior is always a challenge for archaeologists (recall Hawkes's ladder of inference). Yet, with the advent of *Homo erectus* came a new relationship with tools; tools began to enter the social arena, providing a narrow window through which to see the aspects of social cognition.

Settlement patterns, archaeologists' favorite signature for social interaction, are of little help for this phase of human evolution. Ironically, archaeologists know more about settlement patterns of hominins in Phase 1 because they often used spots next to low energy bodies of water that preserved the remains without too much disturbance. *Homo erectus* sites are rarely located in these contexts; more commonly, *Homo erectus* chose sites in higher energy depositional locales, such as the sand beds of intermittent streams. There is very little evidence even for group size for the early part of Phase 2. Indeed, it is not until the lake side occupation of Gesher Benot Ya'aqov (GBY), 780,000 years in age, that archaeologists have anything like a reliable habitation site. Some sites in Africa boast thousands of handaxes concentrated in dense accumulations that do not seem to be entirely the result of water action. Yet, they are not habitation sites or even activity sites. There are a few well-described quarry sites, again mostly late, and as the section on technical cognition mentioned, hominins moved cores and roughouts of tools from quarries to activity sites in a structured way. At GBY itself, the limited lateral extent of the excavations limit direct measures of group size, but the remains suggest a small group that was part of a larger community (Goren-Inbar et al., 2002, 2014, 2018). The weakness of the settlement data means that most interpretations of social cognition rely on analysis of artifacts, with handaxes playing an inordinate role.

Mentalizing, or ToM, plays an important role in human social cognition (Frith & Frith, 2012). Modern people regularly juggle four levels of intentionality in social exchanges (I know that you know that John knows what Robert knows) and sometimes five. How might one track this kind of thing with artifacts? As noted earlier, James Cole (Cole, 2014, 2017; Frith & Frith, 2012) has incorporated some of the perspective of embodied/extended cognition (Malafouris, 2013) to address the role handaxes may have played in communicating information about personal identity. If a stone knapper invested extra effort to produce an exceptional artifact (size, difficult raw material, and thinness), then he or she must have known that others would see it and judge it. And it was not just "others see me." It must have included what others knew about what the maker knew, something akin to "I alter what I do because you know the prototype against which I must conform my efforts. . . . I know that you know that I know." This is third-order intentionality. And if there is a community-wide shared standard, this adds a fourth (Cole, 2014).

Community standards also imply normative rules (Shipton & White, 2020). Much of modern cultural behavior consists of such learned norms, and children begin acquiring them very early in life. Shipton and White report that the basis of such normativity lies in over-imitation: "The developmental basis of normativity is to be found in over-imitation, the uniquely human tendency to replicate all intentional actions of a demonstrator" (article 10232). When human children imitate, they reproduce everything they see about the action, even if it is irrelevant to the result. This quirk leads to arbitrary norms for artifact shapes as novices learn through close observation of what a model or teacher does. The norms for shapes vary from one community of artisans to the next. Shipton and White used a principle component analysis to study handaxe variability in 500,000-year-old sites in Britain and the component that accounted for the most variability was the site of origin. In other words, each community had different set of normative shapes. The variations were unrelated to handaxe function and consisted of different target outlines, differences in how the knappers thinned the tips, and differences in cross-sectional shapes, including "twisted profile" handaxes. Handaxes from the site of Boxgrove (see Fig. 10), which accumulated within a narrow 20- to 80-year period, demonstrate very little variance in shape, and most share the tip thinning techniques known as tranchet. The Boxgrove handaxes have such a uniform target shape that it is possible to recognize slight differences produced by individual knappers (Berlant & Wynn, 2018).

In sum, it appears that by the end of this phase, hominins relied on arbitrary norms in tool manufacture, and by extension, in other components of culture. The over-imitation cited by Shipton and White also required very high-fidelity social learning, with teaching a likely component.

Symbolism and Language

The use of signs is not itself a cognitive ability, but it certainly relies on neural processing and is thus an appropriate target for evolutionary cognitive archaeology. There has, unfortunately, been much sloppy thinking in archaeology about signs and symbols, a sloppiness that would vanish if practitioners relied on a formal system of description derived from semiotics, such as that developed over a century ago by Charles Sanders Peirce (Houser & Kloesel, 1992).

True symbols in his system have an arbitrary link between the sign and what it stands for. They are thus rather difficult to identify in the archaeological record. There is an agreement among archaeologists that modern humans were using symbols extensively by 50,000 years ago. There is little agreement, however, about what went before, or even if true symbols developed out of icons, indexes, or something else entirely. Thirty years ago, Iain Davidson and William Noble (Davidson & Noble, 1989) argued that the use of icons had to have preceded and enabled the emergence of symbols, basing their reasoning in the ecological psychology of James Gibson and Ludwig Wittgenstein's treatment of signs. Archaeological evidence for icons had a very shallow time depth—at the time only about 40,000 years—which led Davidson and Noble to argue further than language was also a very late development. For many scholars of language evolution, such a late date seemed highly unlikely. An alternative archaeological approach to pre-symbolic signs is through indexes, an approach that melds nicely with embodied/extended approaches to cognition.

The interpretant link between an index and what it stands for occurs through extension or association: a hoofprint stands for a deer or smoke stands for fire. There is a natural indexicality to tools; each naturally stands for its use. A firearm is a potent index of its function, for example, and can act effectively even without discharge. Similarly, a stone flake *could* stand for slicing, but to do so it would need to be a potential agent, that is, be a recognized thing. As we discussed earlier, there is no reason to think that the tools of Phase 1 hominins had such status; they were components of procedures and lacked independent status in the minds of the hominins. But handaxes did have such ontological status. The hominins could and did think about them, and their natural indexicality could be exploited.

The FLK West handaxe in Fig. 17 may have acted as such an index. The overdetermination of form and its gigantism exaggerate the toolness of the artifact. Earlier, we suggested that this was an aesthetic effect. It might also have enhanced its indexical effect. Tools not only index their use, they also index their maker. Lambros Malafouris (2008) has made a compelling argument about the Blombos Cave beads (a mere 77,000 years old) in which he suggests that making and wearing personal ornaments enabled the people (*Homo sapiens*) to construct a full concept of self as social agents. We like this argument, but think he places the process far too late in human evolution. Curated, personal tools such as handaxes could have done much the same work. Because the handaxe existed ontologically as an individual tool made by a hominin, it could be an index of him or her by extension, and because they curated these tools, they could cue episodic memories of its previous use and cue prospective memories of its future use, thereby providing temporal extension to the owner. In other words, handaxes were indexes of personal identity.

Over the next 40,000 generations or so, this indexical role of tools slowly accrued more semiotic load. In the 1990s, Kohn and Mithen (1999) suggested that handaxes played a role in sexual selection. Male stone knappers displayed their worth as potential mates by making impressive handaxes. This would be an indexical role, standing for reproductive value. It would not be an arbitrary link because the handaxe is an extension of the artisan. Thus, handaxes were not symbols. Earlier, we discussed Shipton and White's documentation of normativity in British handaxe shapes. Such normative choices index the group of artisans that made them; the tools indexed groups, not just individuals. There is weak corroboration of this role from Boxgrove. The group of *Homo heidelbergensis* that lived there often abandoned handaxes on the edge of a pond, away from any butchery or manufacturing sites, and not associated with a living site. Why? A handaxe might simply have acted as a marker—"I was here," but because the Boxgrove handaxes are all so similar, it would also have marked "we were here," and index that another community could clearly recognize.

Finally, consider these handaxes from Bentadjine in Algeria (Wynn et al., 2020).

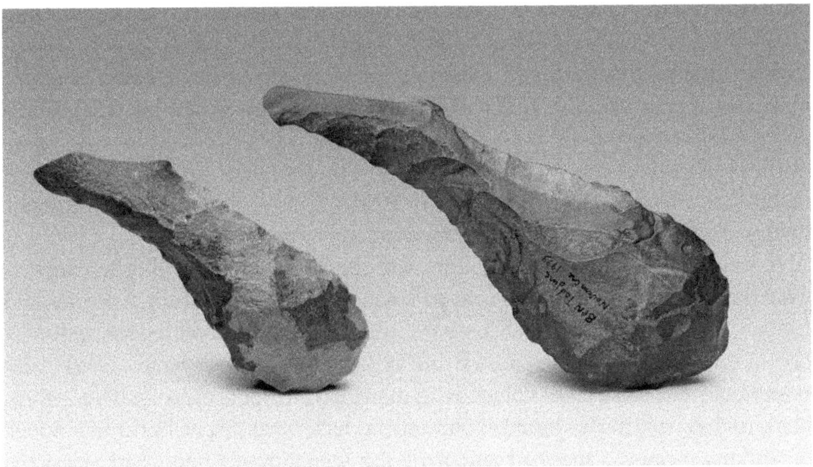

Figure 19 Zoomorphic handaxes from Bentadjine, Algeria, ca. 300,000. Artifact on right is 26 × 8.2 cm. After Berlant and Wynn (2018). With permission of Nasher Sculpture Center.

These two handaxes are zoomorphic, modified to resemble the head and neck of an animal (equid of some kind, perhaps). They are not just indexical, they are iconic. This represents a dramatic expansion of semiotic role. The artifacts refer not just to the maker and the maker's social group, they refer to something that lacks extension or association. These hominins used their artifacts to reference other kinds of things, a giant step toward true symbol use.

The Phase 2 archaeological record reveals nothing about language per se, but given the evidence for social learning, aesthetics, and signs, there are grounds for speculation. The primary components of a language are its words and its grammar. Words are true symbols, and thus, the evidence for a semiotic role for tools is provocative. Indeed, Barham and Everett (2020) have suggested that symbols/words are the only necessary component of language and see the semiotic role of handaxes as adequate evidence for symbolic ability and the presence of words. This is a bold, even iconoclastic stance, and few in the language evolution community would agree. We take a less extreme position. The technical sequences evident at GBY 780,000 years ago imply some kind of teaching, and the variety of procedures and subroutines almost required labels. Thus, we climb part of the way out on the tree limb and suggest that word-based communication was in place by 800 Ka.

Grammar is a more difficult problem. Although it is tempting to liken the complex technical procedures at GBY to sentences, the parallel does not hold up. Modern children learn language and technology very differently, which indicates that they have a different neurological basis. Work by Stout et al.

(Stout & Chaminade, 2012) has confirmed that speech production uses neural resources that initially evolved for object manipulation. This is certainly provocative. Some archaeologists have suggested that hierarchically organized technical procedures are evidence for recursion, a key feature of grammars (Hauser et al., 2002). If this were true, children would learn technical procedures as effortlessly as they learn language. They don't. Moreover, many of these tree structures for technology are artifacts of the analyses; one learns technology mostly sequentially (Wynn, 1991). We see no persuasive argument linking Stone Age technology to grammatical competence.

A word-based oral communication, with perhaps simple word-order rules, is what Bickerton predicted about a proto-language based on his study of pidgins and creoles (Bickerton, 2008). Such a system would be congruent with what archaeology informs us about the hominins living at the end of Phase 2. Simple word-order rules would also make fewer demands upon working memory capacity. Thus, grammar's (or more narrowly syntax) evolution may have been shaped by the limitations of working memory capacity, particularly the limitations of phonological storage (see Coolidge, 2012, for a more detailed explanation for the evolution of grammar).

Change

Phase 2 spanned 1.5 million years, 60,000 generations, and the transition from *Homo erectus* to *Homo heidelbergensis*. It was not a period of stagnation, as archaeologists once thought, but change was excruciatingly slow. To highlight the archaeological evidence for cognitive developments, we arbitrarily pick three salient sign posts—Olduvai Gorge at 1.6 Ma; Gesher Benot Ya'aqov at 780,000 years ago; and Boxgrove at 500,000 years ago.

Olduvai Gorge at 1.6 Ma

Compared to the hominins responsible for Phase 1 sites, the early handaxe makers at Olduvai demonstrate a greater commitment to technology. Associated cognitive developments included:

- A **tool concept.** It is possible that there was only a single, salient, prototype of tool and that other lithics still operated in the context of procedures.
- **Expanded long-term memory**. The technical retrieval structures evident for the FLK West giant required more and longer procedural chains than anything in Phase 1.
- **Expanded working memory**. An increase in cognitive controls, including response inhibition and task switching. Also, there was an enhancement of the **visuospatial sketchpad** of working memory via the coordination of the dorsal and ventral streams of visual processing.
- **Aestheticized tools**. Stone knappers enhanced the visual appeal of artifacts by adhering to good Gestalt forms and using gigantism and other implicit visual effects.

- **Social cognition.** Hominins had second-order intentionality and perhaps third order. Hominins attended to how others viewed their tools, perhaps tied to use in social displays. High-fidelity copying, and perhaps teaching, were necessary for learning technical procedures.
- An **indexical role** for tools that communicated skill and, perhaps, identity.

Gesher Benot Ya'aqov at 780 Ka

Compared to Olduvai Gorge at 1.6 Ma, the hominins at GBY added:

- Multiple, well-delineated **tool types**. The types were linked to separate procedures and almost certainly had different functions.
- **Expanded long-term memory**. Tool production and food processing deployed expert retrieval structures that had more and longer procedural chains and more subroutines. Long-term memory included **episodic memories**.
- **Greater cognitive control**. Evidence for animal and plant processing suggest multielement task switching and the use of **prospective memory**.
- **Aesthetic cognitive** effects included exaggerated prototypicality and use of exceptional raw materials. Rarity of fine examples of handaxes suggests that aesthetics remained in the domain of individual expression. The tools were thus **indexes** of personal identity.
- **Social cognition** included third-order intentionality and teaching.
- **Words** or other declarative reference. The variety and subtle differences between technical procedures would have required labels of some kind. Given that stone knapping uses the hands, any teaching must have used vocal labels.

Boxgrove at 500 Ka

Compared to GBY, the hominins at Boxgrove added:

- **Normative types** that reflected community standards.
- **Allocentric perception** in tool production and probably in navigation as well.
- Social cognition with **fourth-order intentionality**.
- **Indexical reference** for individual and group identity.
- **Proto-language**

Conclusion: A Culture of Expertise

The cognitive component that emerges most clearly from the archaeological record of Phase 2 is expert technical cognition. Expert retrieval structures evolved in capacity via increases in the length and complexity of procedural routines and in the number of routines. This was primarily an expansion of long-term memory capacity, including episodic memory. The working memory component evolved via enhancement in cognitive control and expansion of the visuospatial sketchpad. By the end of Phase 2, expert cognition was a powerful, flexible cognitive strategy that enabled hominins to compete successfully in a large range of habitats in Europe, Asia, and Africa. Indeed, the expert cognition of *Homo heidelbergensis* appears to have been modern in many respects, especially raw capacity. But it was not yet modern. The dearth of innovation tells us that folk theories of causation—the mechanical reasoning of Goldenberg—were either absent or poorly developed. *Homo heidelbergensis* may have had proto-language, but that system had not itself yielded higher level reasoning systems. Today, expert cognition is still an essential component of human success; we rely on it every day for many of our most valued accomplishments. The archaeological record tells us that this form of thinking has very deep roots in the hominin past. But we modern humans are far more creative and inventive than our Phase 2 ancestors. It is this development that is the theme for Phase 3.

14 Phase 3

Emergence of Modern Thinking—300,000–12,000 Years Ago

Phase 3, which lasted about 300,000 years and 12,000 generations, was the shortest and most recent of our divisions of the Palaeolithic. There are far more sites from this phase than the previous two phases combined, and the preservation of these sites is much better. Archaeologists have more data, and better data, including regions with multiple sites of equivalent age. This enables archaeologists to describe activities at a finer scale of resolution. Even if the phase saw no significant evolutionary developments, it would still appear more complex than earlier phases for taphonomic reasons alone. One of the challenges for archaeologists is identifying examples of truly novel of behavior. This phase saw the most recent developments in cognitive abilities, but archaeologists differ vociferously about what, precisely, this entailed, and if the development occurred early in the phase or late. There is also the highly charged issue of the cognitive profile of Neandertals, Denisovans, and other archaic *Homo sapiens* who shared the planet with our ancestors until almost the end of the phase.

Most of the fossil hominin crania dating to Phase 3 have capacities in the modern range [*Homo floresiensis* (Flores Island) and *Homo naledi* (South Africa) are the exceptions]. Indeed, the average *Homo sapiens* cranial capacity appears to have peaked about 100 Ka and has been declining in more recent populations, a phenomenon that we do not understand very well. It may be that the evolution of a more globular brain shape in the modern human line also led to reduced overall volume. It is unclear what implications this has for cognitive ability, though some effect seems likely. Our best record of hominin cognitive abilities remains the archaeological record.

We begin with technical cognition, for it is here that cognitive developments shine through most clearly.

Technical Cognition

The most significant development in technical cognition was the dramatic elaboration of mechanical reasoning. The resources of expert cognition, made up of well-learned procedures held in long-term memory and activated in working memory, had been the hallmarks of technical cognition since the advent handaxes. As long-term memory increased in capacity along with elements of

DOI: 10.4324/9781003014485-17

cognitive control, expertise provided flexibility in problem-solving but little creativity. Innovation was rare in Phases 1 and 2 and probably serendipitous (Wynn & Coolidge, 2014). There is little reason to attribute semantic folk theories of causation to these earlier hominins, but by the middle of Phase 3, our ancestors had begun to think about technical systems in new ways.

Bow and arrow technology is an excellent example. The bow and arrow first appeared in the Middle Stone Age (MSA) of southern Africa between 50 and 100,000 (100 Ka) years ago. Small quartz projectile points from Sibudu were likely arrow points (Lombard & Haidle, 2012) and bone points from other South African MSA sites also appear to have been arrow points (Shea & Sisk, 2010). Using actualistic replication and the ethnographic record of bow and arrow systems in southern Africa, Lombard and Haidle compiled a cognigram of the necessary procedures. It required several pages to present in journal format. Compared to the cognigrams for carving a spear out of spruce (*Homo heidelbergensis* at Schöningen), the bow and arrow cognigram contains many more discrete steps and many more routines and subroutines. Indeed, they found it necessary to separate the system into multiple discrete components (production of stave, production of projectile point, bowstring, adhesive, etc.). The Sibudu hunter or hunters could have executed each component separately in time and space, but all the while they were guided by the overarching project, coordinating the disparate elements. The scope and complexity of this technical system dwarfs the most elaborate systems of Phase 2. The expert retrieval structures that directed the activities required an expansion in long-term memory and enhanced working memory resources. But, more significantly, the resources of expert cognition cannot alone account for the emergence of bow and arrow technology (Coolidge et al. 2016).

The invention of the bow and arrow required minds that were "able to apply abstract engineering concepts" (Gärdenfors & Lombard, 2020, p. 5). Gärdenfors & Lombard base this audacious claim on features of bow and arrow dynamics. Bows work by storing energy in a flexed stave (the bow); when released, the spring back of the stave propels the light projectile. The bow and arrow could not have arisen through small modifications of a preexisting system, such as a thrown spear, or even a spear thrower. The physics is entirely different. Gärdenfors & Lombard suggest it arose after hunters had experience with snares, which are trapping devices based on flexed branches or stalks. The flexed piece stores energy, like a bow. But otherwise, the two technologies are quite different: snares are passive devices that function without direct human action and bows are active hunting machines. For our Stone Age Edison to invent a bow, he or she would have needed to transfer the "physics" from one domain to another. This kind of invention required true creativity based on an abstract understanding of material dynamics.

Gärdenfors & Lombard point to yet another component of bow and arrow hunting that required abstraction—poisons. Arrows are light projectiles that alone cannot reliably kill large mammals. Yet, MSA hunters did kill large mammals such as eland, and even Cape buffalo. How? Modern African hunters and gatherers use poisons. Transferring experience with gustatory poisoning to applying poisons to projectiles required an abstract understanding of folk chemistry. Gärdenfors & Lombard conclude that the MSA bow hunters in southern Africa used abstract causal reasoning (Gardenfors & Lombard, 2018). This conclusion fits nicely with neuroscientist Francois Osiurak's argument for the importance of mechanical reasoning in modern technical cognition:

> The core assumption is that this reasoning is based on *mechanical knowledge* that contains non-declarative. . . , abstract information about physics principles and mechanical actions.
>
> (Osiurak et al., 2020, p. 884). (emphasis in original)

This ability to understand and use abstract ideas about *how* tools work is sometimes labeled "folk physics," and it is a characteristic of all modern human technologies.

Abstract understanding of causality powers invention, which is the most potent vehicle of innovation. Over the long millennia of Phase 2, innovations did accrue, but they were few and very, very far between. The only mechanisms of innovation were serendipitous discoveries based on technical accidents or fiddling about with tools (Wynn & Coolidge, 2014). No one living in Phase 2 had the cognitive resources to intentionally develop a novel technology by applying dynamic relationships inherent in one technology to an unrelated domain, to see "A" in terms of "B." This form of mechanical reasoning was in operation for the invention of the bow and arrow, perhaps 100 Ka. Combined with increased capacity of long-term memory, and enhanced working memory capacity, modern *Homo sapiens* possessed technical problem-solving abilities of almost limitless potential and perhaps for the first time in hominin evolution technology, rather than social life, became the engine driving cognitive evolution.

But abstraction was not limited to technical thinking; it also powered developments in social cognition and symbolic thinking.

Memory

With the better preservation associated with many Phase 3 sites, the evidence for hominin activities expanded significantly, and much of this evidence informs us about long-term memory. Lombard and Haidle's cognigrams of bow and arrow technology describe a dramatic increase in sheer quantity of information compared to even the most complex Phase 2 system (Lombard & Haidle, 2012). This implies a greater long-term memory capacity, but because there is no acceptable metric of long-term memory, this conclusion is little more than a simple comparison of cognigram size. Yet, there is also something episodic about some of the long-term memories in the cognigrams. The bowyer needed not just to remember information, he or she envisioned future scenarios and relied on specific autobiographical memories about sources and events. Better examples come from subsistence activities.

About 65,000 years ago, MSA hunters at Sibudu Cave, South Africa, used traps or snares to hunt blue duiker (Wadley, 2010). The evidence for traps of some kind is indirect but convincing. Blue duiker are small antelope that live in woodlands with dense undergrowth where they move along well-established trails. A hunter could wait by such a trail for a duiker to sprint by, but this would be a poor tactic from a cost-benefit perspective. Modern South African hunters use snares that they set across the trail; this is the only effective means of hunting duiker. In the 65 Ka-levels at Sibudu Cave, the number of duiker remains increased dramatically compared to earlier levels. The hunters must have started using snares or traps. For this kind of trapping to provide a reliable return, it is necessary to maintain and monitor multiple traps—at least ten traps for every person (Janulis, personal communication, February 26, 2019). Such numbers assure that there are enough captures to justify the investment. This is a significant challenge to memory—where the traps are set and when. And, since the hunters set every snare in a similar place (duiker trail), terrain features would provide only modest mnemonic cues. The hunter would need very specific, episodic memories to do this. Such memories were also autobiographical. Indeed, the memory challenge is severe enough that some form of technical assistance may have been necessary, either constructing artificial landmarks to help recall locations, or using a tally system of some sort to keep track of what had been done.

An enhancement of working memory compared to Phase 2 is one of the clearest signatures of Phase 3 (Coolidge & Wynn, 2001, 2005; Wynn & Coolidge, 2010b). We see this both in general demands on the amount of information held in attention and in specific executive functions such as response inhibition, task switching, and control over distance and time. The bow and arrow example and the duiker snare example both implicate enhanced working memory capacity. Manufacturing of adhesives for arrow hafts alone required rapid task switching (Wadley et al., 2009), as did stave and arrow manufacturing. Setting snares relied on inhibition (delayed gratification), and monitoring snares required task switching and prospective memory (Ambrose, 2010). But it was the planning over distance and time that left the most abundant evidence. For example, 40-Ka hunters on Borneo used fire to help manage resources. At Niah Cave, the stratigraphic sequence includes multiple thin ash layers that resulted from local burns of the tropical vegetation (Barker et al., 2007). Such burns led to a "green up" of grasses, which in turn attracted herbivores. This kind of scheduled and managed foraging became common after 100 Ka, and it relied on the resources of enhanced working memory (Coolidge & Wynn, 2005).

Social Cognition

Phase 3 encompassed some of the most significant changes in social behavior ever to occur in hominin evolution. At the beginning of the phase hominins lived in small, mobile hunting and gathering groups loosely allied with other such groups (Dunbar et al., 2014), little different from the Phase 2 hominins who preceded them. By the end of the phase, 12,000 years ago, some *Homo sapiens* lived in sedentary communities with scores, even hundreds of inhabitants. The scale of hominin social interaction expanded dramatically. Clive Gamble, who is the authority on late Palaeolithic social systems, divides this phase into two divisions. In the earlier, 300–60 Ka, hominins increased their range of activities and began to mark social divisions symbolically (Gamble, 1999). In the later division, after 60 Ka, hominins developed ways to establish and maintain far-flung social networks that included acquaintances as well as kin and created elaborate symbolic cultures that unified communities and debarred strangers. This uptick in the scale of social life included the evolution of social cognitive abilities that remain today the basis of modern social cognition. There have been many attempts to characterize these cognitive developments, but we will touch on only a few that we believe have sound archaeological support.

Despite the improvement in preservation and chronological control associated with Phase 3, the interpretation of late Palaeolithic social life remains a challenge. Hawkes's ladder of inference still holds. Settlement patterns are still the primary data sources, but for the earlier chronological division (300–60 Ka), these had not changed much over Phase 2. The archaeological evidence for the sizes of occupation sites is skewed. Most occupation sites in this earlier period are cave sites where preservation and chronological control is good. But most cave sites can accommodate only small groups of people; thus, such sites preserve the residue of small bands of ten to 20 individuals, which in most cases were small foraging groups of a larger community. Larger occupation sites in open terrain rarely preserve. Indeed, it is not until Gamble's second period, after 60 Ka, that archaeologists have any such larger aggregation sites, and most of these post-date 30 Ka. As a consequence, documenting increased social scale rests on three additional varieties of data: geographic range, interaction distance, and regionalization.

Raw material transfers are the primary proxy for geographic range. In a brilliant analysis of European transfer patterns, Gamble (1999) demonstrated that Middle Palaeolithic evidence (300–40 Ka) presented a simple "star-burst" pattern in which raw material moved from sources to central locations, with few examples of transfers over 20 km. The knappers traveled from occupation sites to sources and back home again. The subsequent Aurignacian pattern (40–30 Ka) was a "high-density all-channel" network in which knappers cached high-quality material at some locations and transferred it over successive moves to distant locations, up to several hundred kilometers. The social implications are significant. The Middle Palaeolithic pattern is one of face-to-face groups traveling to sources and returning; no contact with other face-to-face groups is apparent nor was it required. For the Aurignacian pattern, there are two possible social versions. In one, an individual or small group traveled to distant sources, passing through territories of neighboring groups. In the other, socially linked local groups passed raw material from one group to the next, to the next, and so on. In either case, the agents needed to interact with different face-to-face groups, a clear extension of the range of social contacts and interaction. A similar pattern emerged in the Balkans at about the same time. At the Romanian site of Poiana Cireşului, archaeologists recovered beads made of *Homalopoma sanguineum* shells, a Mediterranean mollusk whose nearest possible source was 900 km distant (Niţul et al., 2019). Once again, either the residents of Poiana Cireşului traveled themselves to the Mediterranean coast, in which case they needed to pass through territories of possible hostile groups, or they traded for these items via a trade network.

By 30 Ka, there were much larger habitation sites, suggesting larger face-to-face groups. The 30 Ka complex of sites at Dolní Věstonice-Pavlov in the Czech Republic is an excellent example (Gamble, 1999; Svoboda, 2020). The inhabitants build substantial oval huts, each about 5 m in diameter and often anchored with mammoth bone. These were large enough for a family group of five to ten. Each hut had a central hearth and pits for storage. Population estimates for total group size suggest scores of inhabitants, perhaps as many as 100 (Svoboda, 2020, p. 159). Site evidence includes huge deposits of mammoth bone bordering the occupation area, a large open central hearth, burials with grave goods, and the earliest known fired ceramic figurines, including the famous "Black Venus." The site was occupied for much of the year, perhaps even year-round. Not only was the site larger, it was internally differentiated with specialized activity areas. Dolní Věstonice-Pavlov is unusual for its level of preservation and variety of evidence, but other contemporary sites such as Abri Pataud in France corroborate many of its features, including group size and internal differentiation of activity areas (Gamble, 1999).

By 30 Ka, people were marking their group identity with explicit artifact styles. These included styles of tool manufacture and ornament production that were practiced by one community but not by their neighbors. Belfer-Cohen and Hovers (Belfer-Cohen & Hovers, 2020) have documented the development of such distinctive styles soon after 40 Ka in the Levant. Communities in what is today Northern Israel made a distinctive ornament by carving notches in the scapulae of gazelle. Neighboring groups did not make such artifacts, and thus, the notched bones were emblematic of this community. Belfer-Cohen and Hovers suggest that such community styles marked the maintenance of socio-cultural boundaries and the emergence of "others" as an ontological category in the social universe.

Mortuary treatment is another piece to the puzzle of Phase 3 social life. Archaeologists often discuss mortuary treatment as a component of symbolic behavior, but there are also social implications. The earliest evidence for mortuary treatment is the site of Sima de los Huesos, at Atapuerca in Spain, which dates to the end of Phase 2 (>400 Ka). This "pit of bones" is a shaft inside a cave down which hominins deposited 30 corpses (Pettitt, 2013). Archaeologists found one handaxe in association, but this may have been an accidental loss. Later, in Phase 3, Neandertals often protected corpses by covering them with large stones or digging shallow graves, though this was far from universal. There are no convincing examples of grave goods. Similarly, early modern humans also dug graves for corpses and occasionally included grave goods. After 30 Ka, some of these graves, such as those at Sunghir in Russia, included elaborate grave goods with beads and weapons (Trinkaus & Buzhilova, 2018). This mortuary evidence provides clues to social behavior. First, they corroborate the extension of social life. Even the enigmatic Sima de los Huesos suggests that the dead continued to have social agency after death. This does not require an abstract notion of afterlife; it could have been simply memories of the dead influencing the actions of the living. Second, after 30 Ka, differences in mortuary treatment suggest social differentiation within communities. At Sunghir, two of the burials were juveniles interred with thousands of ivory beads, which suggests an inherited position of rank.

It is important to reiterate that archaeological arguments about social cognition require an initial inference about social behavior and thus tend to be more tentative than the conclusions about technical cognition. We believe that the evidence comfortably supports two conclusions about Phase 3 trends in social life: First, social extension increased to include more individuals in face-to-face groups, maintenance of social links to other communities and eventually strangers, and temporal extension of social roles beyond death. Second, evidence supports increasing community differentiation of activities and roles. What cognitive developments accompanied these trends?

Frith and Frith (2012) emphasized the importance of explicit, top-down cognitive processes when they contrasted human social cognition with that of other primates. Much of human social cognition continues to rely on implicit processes whose features evolved out of homologous abilities shared with other primates. For example, human Theory of Mind evolved out of primate level precursors such as gaze following. ToM is still a largely implicit process whose scope evolved over the course of human evolution. But at some point, humans acquired meta-cognitive abilities that enabled them to reflect on their mental states—to think about thinking and manipulate this knowledge. According to Firth and Firth, this meta-cognitive ability enabled people to suspend or overcome strong implicit biases in social cognition. One of these is fear of outgroups—communities that are not one's own. If one can suppress this pre-attentive hostility, one can negotiate with acquaintances and strangers, thus dramatically expanding one's social network. Related to this is the ability to share experiences. If one can listen to another's autobiographical memories and learn from them, one increases one's knowledge of important information about resources, dangers, and changing conditions. It also increases the effectiveness of teaching. These all require meta-cognition—thinking about pre-attentive social responses (fear of outgroup), about another's memories (sharing experience) and abilities (teaching). Such social meta-cognition resembles, of course, the mechanical knowledge component of technical cognition, whose folk physics consists of reflections on the nature of tool-linked causality. Such top-down reflection on cognitive states takes place in working memory and thus enhanced working memory was one of the prerequisites for these developments (Coolidge & Wynn 2005).

Aesthetic Cognition

Phase 3 witnessed an increase in the number, variety, and sophistication of aesthetic productions and performances, especially after 100 Ka. We include in this category personal ornaments, decorative patterns and treatments, body decoration and alteration, and representational and symbolic images such as figurines and rock art. Most abundant are the ornaments, which derive from sites throughout Eurasia and, after 50 Ka, Australia. The earliest consist of marine shells punctured and strung as necklaces or pendants, but other natural items quickly followed, including animal teeth. Eventually, after 50 Ka, people invested more effort in the manufacture of ornaments out of bone, antler, and ivory. The "basket" beads of the European Aurignacian (ca. 40–30 Ka) were carved from mammoth ivory, punctured with a stone tool, polished, and strung onto necklaces. Each bead required several hours of labor (Gamble, 1999). At Sunghir in Russia (also ca. 30 Ka), the mortuary treatments included thousands of similar ivory beads, which appear to have adorned clothing. People also decorated their everyday artifacts. Geometric patterns were popular, including cross-hatchings, slashes, and zones of dots. Some of these patterns occurred in multiple sites, attesting to local conventions and traditions. Justly famous are the examples of rock art, examples of which occur on every continent. People adorned rock walls and boulders with engraved (petroglyphs) and painted (pictographs) patterns and images. Sometimes people produced not only images of animals but also enigmatic geometric patterns. Positive and negative handprint pictographs were also common.

The Phase 2 impulse to overdetermine the form of artifacts continued in Phase 3. The same basic Gestalt forms and implicit visual effects characterize the aesthetic products of this phase, and indeed many examples of "symbolic" artifacts are more easily explained through these more ancient aesthetic components (Hodgson, 2014). But Phase 3 aesthetics also incorporated that elusive fourth component of aesthetic cognition—investing aesthetic production with cultural values and symbolic meanings. This drew on not only the pre-attentive components of aesthetic cognition but also personal and cultural memories and explicit references to abstract concepts, as with the Hohlenstein-Stadel therianthrope. Put differently, Phase 3 saw the development of art as we currently know and experience it.

Modern *Homo sapiens* appear to have been the primary, but not the only, Palaeolithic artists. They were responsible for most of the examples listed previously. Neandertals did use body decorations, including coloring and use of feathers. There are also a handful of Neandertal-produced pendants. This appears to have been an independent development out of local European Phase 2 aesthetics. It never approached the level of investment seen with modern humans after 50 Ka, who truly seem to have immersed themselves in aesthetic performances. The earliest musical instruments (swan-bone flutes) were made by the same people who made the Hohlenstein-Stadel figurine, 40,000 years ago (d'Errico et al., 2003).

Symbolism

One of the distinctive characteristics of the Phase 3 archaeological record is the dramatic increase in evidence for semiotic activities. Some of this trend reflects the better preservation and higher survival rates for more recent sites. Preservation of organic material other than bone expanded the range of artifacts available to archaeologists for interpretation, including objects with semiotic implications. But the trend also appears to reflect a real increase in the number and variety of semiotic activities practiced by Palaeolithic people. Current evidence divides the phase into three chronological periods. Evidence from 300 to 100 Ka offers only scattered, isolated examples of possible semiotic activity—the Twin Rivers ochre or the Bentadjine zoomorphic bifaces. These suggest that people were occasionally producing artifacts with semiotic "load," but always via indexical or iconic reference in the Peircean sense. From 100 to 50 Ka in Africa, there was a significant uptick in semiotic evidence. Beads and engraved ochre pieces from Blombos Cave attest to possible indexical marking (Henshilwood & Dubreuil, 2011) and fragments of engraved ostrich eggshells from a variety of sites point to a decorative tradition. There is also now sound evidence from this period that Neandertals made and used pendants. None of this is convincingly symbolic in the Peircean sense, but its expansion fits well with the expanded social lives indicated by the movement of raw material. People now had reason to mark their social affiliations. Evidence for true symbols does not appear until after 50 Ka, and so far, the evidence points to modern *Homo sapiens* as its primary agent.

Earlier in the text, we discussed several examples of true symbolic artifacts—the Hohlenstein-Stadel figurine and geometric cave paintings. Here, we would like to emphasize an artifact type that we find especially provocative because it implicates not just symbol use, but abstract meta-cognition. These are the "tally" boards or sticks.

The Tai Plaque is a flat piece of bone engraved with hundreds of lines and slash marks. It is about 14,000 years old (Marshack, 1991; d'Errico, 2001). The maker was apparently using the artifact to record something, using the slashes as tallies and the long lines as a frame to maintain a kind of order to

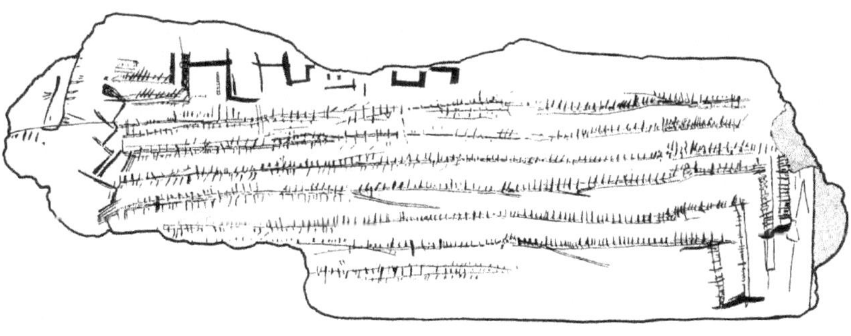

Figure 20 Tai Plaque, 8.8 cm, ca. 14,000 BP, after (Marshack, 1991).

accumulating marks. It appears to be a material aid to quantification. Counting is based on one-to-one correspondence—for example, one reindeer, one slash. We can train chimpanzees to do something like it, but it takes many experimental repetitions, and at best, chimpanzees are limited to about five items (Matsuzawa, 2001). Finger counting is very common worldwide, though not universal, and is based on one-to-one correspondence. It does not require a true number concept; for example, two-hands-worth of fingers is more than one-hands-worth. Finger counting is a definite improvement over magnitude comparison (this group is larger than that), but one soon runs out of body parts. This is when artifacts become essential. They enable the extension of tallying beyond the body part capacity. More provocatively, as Overmann has convincingly argued (Overmann, 2016, 2017), such artifacts acted as the material scaffold for the invention of abstract numbers. One feature of numbers is cardinality ($1 + 1 = 2; 2 + 1 = 3; n+1=x$), which is an abstract principle that needed to be invented. But how did anyone invent such an abstract principle? Without some real-world phenomena, one could never discover relations that suggested a general abstract rule. Tally boards (or knotted strings or strings of beads) provided a material pattern that enabled people to think about quantities and invent a rule of cardinality [and ordinality (Wynn et al., 2017)].

The Tai plaque is an excellent example, but it is not the earliest. Similar artifacts with slashes, dots, or notches date back at least 30 Ka in Europe. Not all engraved objects qualify as quantification devices. Sometimes people decorated objects with these patterns for aesthetic reasons. Distinguishing between the two is a challenge. If the archaeologist can discern that different engraving tools made different sets of marks in separate episodes (d'Errico & Cacho, 1994), then decoration becomes the less likely of the two explanations. Using this standard, d'Errico et al. have recognized notational devices as old 30 Ka.

Tallying devices are important to reconstructions of Phase 3 cognition for two reasons. First, they reinforce the role of meta-cognition, and second, they document the importance of extended cognition. One can discover the cardinal principle only if one thinks about counting, which itself is a form of attentional thinking. This is meta-cognition, akin to thinking about tool manipulation and thinking about social relations, evident in other components of Phase 3 life. All this "thinking about" was a challenge for working memory capacity and, not surprisingly, evidence points to an expansion of working memory capacity over the course of Phase 3. *Homo sapiens* also offloaded some of this capacity onto objects. D'Errico has described tally boards as "external memory devices," but they were a bit more than this. They not only offloaded information, they enabled a manipulation of information and, as Overmann has demonstrated, they led to the invention of abstract concepts. This reliance on objects for thinking becomes a motif for all subsequent developments in human cognition.

Language

It is difficult to imagine how inventions of abstract principles could have occurred in the absence of language, and most scholars are comfortable attributing fully modern language abilities to modern humans who lived after 50 Ka. However, this is a conclusion of convenience, not a well-grounded inference. Moreover, it typically excludes other Phase 3 populations of *Homo sapiens* such as Neandertals, exacerbating the already fraught debate about the nature and fate of these very near cousins. Neandertals, it seems, must prove their case for inclusion in the language-using club. Rudolf Botha (2020) has written a closely reasoned and thoroughly documented discussion of the arguments for Neandertal language, and there are many. He found that they all fall short of his standard for well-reasoned inferences about the past (a standard, readers will recall, that guides this text as well). The strongest of these weak arguments was circumstantial, suggesting that Neandertals must have had some form of linguistic communication to arrange for and execute cooperative hunts, which are a well-attested feature of Neandertal life. The problem with the almost universal attribution of language to post-50 Ka modern humans is that it, too, is entirely circumstantial. Arguments for modern *Homo sapiens* language based on the 77 Ka Blombos beads (d'Errico et al., 2005) are no better grounded and warranted than arguments for Neandertal language (Botha, 2006).

Nevertheless, the circumstantial evidence for language is abundant for modern *Homo sapiens*, especially after 50 Ka. The evidence for material symbols is compelling evidence for fully modern semiotic ability. Objects such as the Hohlenstein-Stadel figurine required an ability to manipulate semiotic reference and conceive of abstract relations. The arbitrary link between words and meaning is simple in comparison. Thus, the circumstantial evidence for words is strong. Evidence for syntax is, as always, more elusive. However, the folk physics of mechanical reasoning and invention and the abstract relations inherent in some material symbols would be difficult to communicate and learn without syntax, but perhaps not impossible.

Neandertals

Neandertals were a branch of *Homo sapiens* who evolved in northwestern Eurasia after 500 Ka and disappeared as a distinct population soon after an influx of African *Homo sapiens* that began sometime before 50 Ka. Since their discovery and description in the 1850s, they have been consistently fascinating to the public and they have become the only fossil hominins to have entered the common vernacular. Everyone, it seems, has some familiarity with Neandertals, if not an accurate knowledge of the evidence. From the vantage point of overall hominin evolution, they do not warrant such special affection. They were a peripheral population that contributed comparatively little to the line of descent leading to modern populations and, like many such populations in the evolutionary past, passed into extinction. However, they did contribute some alleles to the modern gene pool and, more importantly, they are far and away the best documented group of *Homo sapiens* other than modern humans. Science knows a great deal about them because they lived during Phase 3, when preservation was good, and they lived in Europe, where archaeologists have been excavating sites and skeletons for 150 years.

How different were Neandertals? The fossil evidence presents modest but clear differences in postcranial and cranial anatomy. Neandertal skulls had larger faces and larger brain cases; indeed, their average cranial capacity (ca. 1,450–1,550 cc) exceeds that of living *Homo sapiens*. The brain cases were also shaped a bit differently, being longer, with the position of maximum breadths situated lower on the calvarium. Reconstructions of Neandertal brains based on endocasts and sophisticated imaging systems indicate that they were also shaped differently from those of living *Homo sapiens*. Neandertals had relatively smaller parietal lobes, larger occipital lobes, and smaller cerebella. Archaic DNA from Neandertal skeletons includes genes for brain development that differ slightly from their modern *Homo sapiens* counterparts (Gregory et al., 2017). Given these brain differences, it is reasonable to hypothesize that there was a cognitive difference as well. Such a hypothesis can be checked against the archaeological record, making an account of Neandertal cognition an interesting test of the methods of evolutionary cognitive archaeology.

The archaeological evidence points to a modest difference between Neandertal cognition and that of modern *Homo sapiens*. In most respects, the archaeological signatures of Neandertals and African *Homo sapiens* of equivalent age are very similar (Wynn et al., 2016). They both lived in small hunting and gathering communities and exploited a variety of local plants and animals. Both were successful cooperative hunters able to kill and process large mammals. Both also relied on plants and smaller animals and fish. Their technologies were similar. Both used sophisticated stone knapping procedures, hafted stone points onto spear shafts, and made and maintained fire. Both cared for sick and injured group members, and both practiced mortuary treatment. Indeed, Neandertals and African *Homo sapiens* present a similar picture of well-developed expert technical and social systems. Differences did not emerge until after 100 Ka, and they were small, but perhaps ultimately significant. African *Homo sapiens* invented the bow-and-arrow, which as we have seen required a folk physics that included knowledge of dynamic properties of materials. There is nothing comparable in Neandertal technology. African *Homo sapiens* developed trapping systems for small game that operated without human attendants, but which required expanded working memory capacity and an ability to organize episodic memories. African *Homo sapiens*' use of ornaments rapidly developed into a heavier investment in number and variety of aesthetic and semiotic objects. All these point to a greater engagement of meta-cognition by African *Homo sapiens* after 100 Ka, a cognitive profile that differed from that of Neandertals. This difference might have tipped the balance toward modern *Homo sapiens* when the two encountered one another in Eurasia about 50,000 years ago.

Conclusion

This summary of hominin cognitive evolution is brief and tentative. The details will undoubtedly change as cognitive archaeologists apply more and better theories and methods to the evidence at hand, and to new discoveries. Some of our conclusions will survive further testing and research, but others will prove to be incomplete, misguided, or just plain wrong. This is the nature of scientific enquiry. We are confident, however, that evolutionary cognitive archaeology will continue to provide compelling accounts of the evolution of the human mind.

Epilogue

At the beginning of this brief introduction, we aligned evolutionary cognitive archaeology with the realist camp in the history and philosophy of science. In Section I, we tried to show how, with appropriate archaeological data and sound, theoretically grounded inferences, it is possible to describe real features of hominin cognition in the deep past. We acknowledged in Section II, however, that evolutionary cognitive archaeologists have reliable access to only a narrow range of cognitive domains. Comprehensive descriptions of the cognitive life of early hominins are effectively out of reach. There is much we will never know. Yet, there is much that we can know. The archaeological record provides the only direct evidence of past hominin activities that science possesses. If one is interested in the evolution of the human mind, evolutionary cognitive archaeology is the logical place to begin. The 3.3-million-year archaeological record and the cognitive inferences it supports provide a solid scaffold on which other approaches to cognitive evolution, such as paleoneurology and evolutionary psychology, can frame their interpretations.

References

Abramiuk, M. (2012). *The foundations of cognitive archaeology*. MIT Press.

Abramson, C. I., & Chicas-Mosier, A. M. (2016). Learning in plants: Lessons from *Mimosa pudica*. *Frontiers in Psychology*, *7*, Article 417.

Allen, T. A., & Fortin, N. J. (2013). The evolution of episodic memory. *Proceedings of the National Academy of Sciences*, *110*(Supplement 2), 10379–10386.

Alperson-Afil, N., Goren-Inbar, N., Herzlinger, G., & Wynn, T. (2020). Expert retrieval structures and prospective memory in the cognition of Acheulian hominins. *Psychology*, *11*, 173–189.

Ambrose, S. (2010). Coevolution of composite-tool technology, constructive memory, and language: Implications for the evolution of modern human behavior. In T. Wynn & F. Coolidge (Eds.), *Working memory: Beyond language and symbolism* (pp. S135–S147). University of Chicago Press.

Andouze, F., & Karlin, C. (2017). 70 years of "chaine operatoire": What French prehistorians have done with it [La chaine operatoire a 70 ans: Qu'en ont fair les prehistoriens francais]. *Journal of Lithic Studies*, *4*(2), 1–69.

Arbib, M. A., & Bickerton, D. (Eds.). (2010). *The emergence of protolanguage: Holophrasis vs compositionality* (Vol. 24). John Benjamins Publishing.

Atran, S. (1990). *Cognitive foundations of natural history: Towards an anthropology of science*. Cambridge University Press.

Baddeley, A. D. (2001). Is working memory still working? *American Psychologist*, 56(11), 851–864.

Baddeley, A. D. (2007). *Working memory, thought, and action*. Oxford University Press.

Baddeley, A. D. (2012). Working memory: Theories, models, and controversies. *Annual Review of Psychology*, 63, 1–29.

Baddeley, A. D., & Hitch, G. (1974). Working memory. *Psychology of Learning and Motivation*, 8, 47–89.

Barham, L. (2002). Systematic pigment use in the middle Pleistocene of South-Central Africa. *Current Anthropology*, 43(1), 181–190.

Barham, L., & Everett, D. (2020). Semiotics and the origins of language in the lower Palaeolithic. *Journal of Archaeological Method & Theory*. doi:10.1007/s10816-020-09480-9

Barker, G., Barton, H., Bird, M., Daly, P., Datan, I., Dykes, A., Farr, L., Gilbertson, D., Harrisson, B., Hunt, C., Higham, T., Kealhofer, L., Krigbaum, J., Lewis, H., McLaren, S., Paz, V., Pike, A., Piper, P., Pyatt, B., & Turney, C. (2007). The "human revolution" in lowland tropical Southeast Asia: The antiquity and behaviour of anatomically modern humans at Niah Cave (Sarawak, Borneo). *Journal of Human Evolution*, 52, 243–261.

Barnard, P. (2010). From executive mechanisms underlying perception and action to the parallel processing of meaning. *Current Anthropology*, *52*(S1), S39–S54.

Belfer-Cohen, A., & Hovers, E. (2020). Prehistoric perspectives on "others" and "strangers". *Frontiers in Psychology: Conceptual Analysis*, *10*, Article 3083. doi:10 3389/fpsyg 201903083

Berlant, T., & Wynn, T. (2018). *First sculpture: Handaxe to figure stone*. Nasher Sculpture Center.

Bickerton, D. (2008). *Bastard tongues: A trailblazing linguist finds clues to our common humanity in the world's lowliest languages*. Hill and Wang.

Bolhuis, J. J., Tattersall, I., Chomsky, N., & Berwick, R. C. (2014). How could language have evolved? *PLoS Biology*, *12*(8), e1001934.

Botha, R. (2006). *Theoretical underpinnings of inferences about language evolution*. Paper presented at the Cradle of Language, Stellenbosch, South Africa.

Botha, R. (2016). *Language evolution: The windows approach*. Cambridge University Press.

Botha, R. (2020). *Neanderthal language: Demystifying the linguistic powers of our extinct cousins*. Cambridge University Press.

Braun, D., Harris, J., & Maina, D. (2009). Oldowan raw material procurement and use: Evidence from the Koobi Fora formation. *Archaeometry*, *51*, 26–42.

Bronfman, Z. Z., Ginsburg, S., & Jablonka, E. (2016). The transition to minimal consciousness through the evolution of associative learning. *Frontiers in Psychology*, *7*, Article 1954.

Brown, S., Gao, X., Tisdelle, L., Eickhoff, S., & Liotti, M. (2011). Naturalizing aesthetics: Brain areas for aesthetic appraisal across sensory modalities. *Neuroimage*, *58*, 250–258. doi:10.1016/j.neuroimage.2011.06.012

Bruner, E. (2004). Geometric morphometrics and paleoneurology: Brain shape evolution in the genus Homo. *Journal of Human Evolution*, *47*(5), 279–303.

Bruner, E. (Ed.). (2015). *Human paleoneurology*. Springer.

Buss, D. (2003). *The evolution of desire: Strategies of human mating*. Basic Books.

Byrne, R., & Whiten, A. (Eds.). (1988). *Machiavellian intelligence: Social expertise and the evolution of intellect in monkeys, apes, and humans*. Clarendon Press.

Carey, S. (2009). *The origin of concepts*. Oxford University Press.

Chatterjee, A. (2014). *The aesthetic brain: How we evolved to desire beauty and enjoy art*. Oxford University Press.

Chazan, M. (2017). Toward a long prehistory of fire. *Current Anthropology*, 58, S351–S359.

Cole, J. (2014). The identity model: A theory to access visual display and hominin cognition within the Palaeolithic. In R. Dunbar, C. Gamble, & J. Gowlett (Eds.), *Lucy to language: The benchmark papers*. Oxford University Press.

Cole, J. (2017). Accessing hominin cognition: Language and social signalling in the lower to middle palaeolithic. In T. Wynn & F. L. Coolidge (Eds.), *Cognitive models in palaeolithic archaeology* (pp. 157–196). Oxford University Press.

Conard, N. J. (2003). Palaeolithic ivory sculptures from southwestern Germany and the origins of figurative art. *Nature*, *426*, 830–832.

Coolidge, F. L. (1974/2015). *Memory consolidation as function of sleep and the circadian rhythm*. Andesite Press.

Coolidge, F. L. (2012). On the emergence of grammatical language as a means of bypassing the limitations of working memory capacity. *Physics of Life Reviews*, 9, 217–218.

Coolidge, F. L., Haidle, M. N., Lombard, M., & Wynn, T. (2016). Bridging theory and bow hunting: Human cognitive evolution and archaeology. *Antiquity*, 90, 219–228.

Coolidge, F. L., & Wynn, T. (2001). Executive functions of the frontal lobes and the evolutionary ascendancy of *Homo sapiens*. *Cambridge Archaeological Journal*, *11*, 255–260.

Coolidge, F. L., & Wynn, T. (2005). Working memory, its executive functions, and the emergence of modern thinking. *Cambridge Archaeological Journal*, *15*(1), 5–26.

Coolidge, F. L., & Wynn, T. (2006). The effects of the tree-to-ground sleep transition in the evolution of cognition in early *Homo*. *Before Farming*, *2006*, Article 11, 1–18.

Coolidge, F. L. & Wynn, T. (2009, September). Did Neandertals lack diplomatic speech? Cognitive prerequisites for speaking indirectly. *Evolution of Brain, Behavior, & Intelligence Conference*. Wellcome Trust Centre, Hinxton, UK.

Cosmides, L. (1989). The logic of social exchange: Has natural selection shaped how humans reason? Studies with the Wason selection task. *Cognition*, *31*, 187–276.

Currie, G., & Zhu, X. (2021). Aesthetic sense and social cognition: A story from the early stone age. *Synthese*, *198*, 6553–6572.

Davidson, I. (2010). The colonization of Australia and its adjacent islands and the evolution of modern cognition. *Current Anthropology*, *51* (Supplement 1), S177–S189.

Davidson, I., & Noble, W. (1989). The archaeology of perception: Traces of depiction and language. *Current Anthropology*, *30*, 125–155.

Davidson, I., & Noble, W. (1992). Why the first colonisation of the Australian region is the earliest evidence of modern human behaviour. *Archaeology in Oceania*, *27*, 135–142.

Davidson, I., & Noble, W. (1993). Tools and language in human evolution. In K. Gibson & T. Ingold (Eds.), *Tools, language, and cognition in human evolution* (pp. 263–288). Cambridge University Press.

Dehaene, S., & Cohen, L. (2007). Cultural recycling of cortical maps. *Neuron*, *56*, 384–398.

Delagnes, A., & Roche, H. (2005). Late Pliocene hominid knapping skills: The case of Lokalalei 2C, West Turkana, Kenya. *Journal of Human Evolution*, *48*, 435–472.

d'Errico, F. (2001). Memories out of mind: The archaeology of the oldest memory systems. In A. Nowell (Ed.), *In the mind's eye: Multidisciplinary approaches to the evolution of human cognition* (pp. 33–49). International Monographs in Prehistory.

d'Errico, F., & Cacho, C. (1994). Notation versus decoration in the upper Palaeolithic: A case study from Tossal de la Roca, Alicante, Spain. *Journal of Archaeological Science*, *21*, 185–200.

d'Errico, F., Henshilwood, C., Lawson, G., Vanhaeren, M., Tillier, A. M., Soressi, M., Bresson, F., Maureille, B., Nowell, A., Lakarra, J., Backwell, L., & Julien, M. (2003). Archaeological evidence for the emergence of language, symbolism, and music—an alternative multidisciplinary perspective. *Journal of World Prehistory*, *17*(1), 1–70.

d'Errico, F., Henshilwood, C., Vanhaeren, M., & van Niekerk, K. (2005). *Nassarius kraussianus* shell beads from Blombos cave: Evidence for symbolic behaviour in the middle stone age. *Journal of Human Evolution*, *48*, 3–24.

d'Errico, F., Vanhaeren, M., & Wadley, L. (2008). Possible shell beads from the middle stone age layers of Sibudu Cave, South Africa. *Journal of Archaeological Science*, *35*, 2675–2685.

Diez-Martin, F., Wynn, T., Sanchez-Yustos, P., Duque, J., Fraile, C., de Francisco, S., Uribelarrea, D., Mabulla, A., Baquedano, E., & Dominguez-Rodrigo, M. (2019). A faltering origin for the Acheulean? Technological and cognitive implications from FLK West (Olduvai Gorge, Tanzania). *Quaternary International*, *526*, 49–66.

d'Isa, R., Solari, N., & Brambilla, R. (2011). Biological memory in animals and in man. In G. Campardo, F. Tiziani, & M. Iaculo (Eds.), *Memory mass storage* (pp. 417–441). Springer.

Dunbar, R. (1993). Coevolution of neocortical size, group and language in humans. *Behavioral and Brain Sciences*, *16*, 681–735.

Dunbar, R. (1998). The social brain hypothesis. *Evolutionary Anthropology*, *6*, 178–190.

Dunbar, R., Barrett, L., & Lycett, J. (2005). *Evolutionary psychology: A beginner's guide*. Oneworld.

Dunbar, R., Gamble, C., & Gowlett, J. (2010). *Social brain, distributed mind*. British Academy.

Dunbar, R., Gamble, C., & Gowlett, J. (Eds.). (2014). *Lucy to language: The benchmark papers*. Oxford University Press.

Ericsson, K., & Delaney, P. (1999). Long-term working memory as an alternative to capacity models of working memory in everyday skilled performance. In A. Miyake & P. Shah (Eds.), *Models of working memory: Mechanisms of active maintenance and executive control* (pp. 257–297). Cambridge University Press.

Fiske, A. P. (2004). Four modes of constituting relationships: Consubstantial assimilation; space, magnitude, time, and force; concrete procedures; abstract symbolism. In N. Haslam (Ed.), *Relational models theory: A contemporary overview*. Lawrence Erlbaum.

Fitch, W., Hauser, M., & Chomsky, N. (2005). The evolution of the language faculty: Clarification and implications. *Cognition*, *97*(2), 179–210.

Frith, C., & Frith, U. (2012). Mechanisms of social cognition. *Annual Review of Psychology*, *63*, 287–313.

Gamble, C. (1999). *The palaeolithic societies of Europe*. Cambridge University Press.

Gärdenfors, P., & Högberg, A. (2017). The archaeology of teaching and the evolution of *Homo docens*. *Current Anthropology*, *58*(2), 188–208.

Gardenfors, P., & Lombard, M. (2018). Causal cognition, force dynamics and early hunting technologies. *Frontiers in Psychology*, *9*, 87.

Gardenfors, P., & Lombard, M. (2020). Technology led to more abstract causal reasoning. *Biology and Philosophy*, *35*(4), 40.

Gilbert, J. (2018). *The forgotten transition: From event to object and from tool to language*. Gompel & Svacina.

Gladwin, T. (1970). *East is a big bird*. Harvard University Press.

Gobet, F. (2016). *Understanding expertise: A multi-disciplinary approach*. Palgrave.

Goldenberg, G. (2012). Effects of brain damage on human tool use. In T. McCormack, C. Hoerl, & S. Butterfill (Eds.), *Tool use and causal cognition*. Oxford University Press.

Goldenberg, G., & Spatt, J. (2009). The neural basis of tool use. *Brain*, *132*, 1645–1655.

Golomb, C. (1992). *The child's creation of a pictorial world*. University of California Press.

Goren-Inbar, N., Alperson-Afil, N., Sharon, G., & Herzinger, G. (2018). *The acheulian site of Gesher Benot Ya'aqov Volume IV: The lithic assemblages*. Springer.

Goren-Inbar, N., Melamed, Y., Zohar, I., Akhilesh, K., & Pappu, S. (2014). Beneath still waters—multistage aquatic exploitation of euryale ferox (Salisb.) during the Acheulian. *Internet Archaeology*, *37*.

Goren-Inbar, N., Werker, E., & Feibel, C. S. (2002). *The acheulian site of Gesher Benot Ya'aqov, Israel: The wood assemblage*. Oxbow Books.

Gowlett, J. (2006). The elements of design form in Acheulian bifaces: Modes, modalities, rules and language. In N. Goren-Inbar & G. Sharon (Eds.), *Axe age: Acheulian toolmaking from quarry to discard* (pp. 203–222). Equinox.

Greenfield, P. (1991). Language, tools, and brain: The ontogeny and phylogeny of hierarchically organized sequential behavior. *Behavioral and Brain Sciences*, *14*, 531–595.

Gregory, M., Kippenhan, S., Eisenberg, D., Kohn, P., Dickinson, D., Mattay, V., Chen, Q., Weinberger, D. R., Saad, Z. S., & Berman, K. (2017). Neanderthal-derived genetic variation shapes modern cranium and brain. *Nature Scientific Reports*, *7*, 6308. doi:10.1038/s41598-017-06587-0

Guida, A., Gobet, F., Tardieu, H., & Nicolas, S. (2012). How chunks, long-term working memory and templates offer a cognitive explanation for neuroimaging data on expertise acquisition: A two-stage framework. *Brain and Cognition*, *79*, 221–244.

Haidle, M. (2009). How to think a simple spear. In S. De Baune, F. Coolidge, & T. Wynn (Eds.), *Cognitive archaeology and human evolution* (pp. 57–74). Cambridge University Press.

Haidle, M. (2010). Working-memory capacity and the evolution of modern cognitive potential. *Current Anthropology*, *51* (Supplement 1), S149–S166.

Harmand, S., Lewis, J., Feibel, C. S., Lepre, C., Prat, S., Lenoble, A., Boës, X., Quinn, R.L., Brenet, M., Arroyo, A., & Roche, H. (2015). 3.3-million-year-old stone tools from Lomekwi 3, West Turkana, Kenya. *Nature*, *521*, 310–315.

Hauser, M., Chomsky, N., & Fitch, W. (2002). The faculty of language: What is it, who has it, and how did it evolve? *Science*, *298*, 1569–1579.

Hawkes, C. (1954). Archeological theory and method: Some suggestions from the old world. *American Anthropologist*, *56*, 155–168.

Hecht, E., Gutman, D., Kreisheh, N., Taylor, S., Kilner, J., Faisal, A., Bradley, B. A., Chaminade, T., & Stout, D. (2014). Acquisition of Paleolithic toolmaking abilities involves structural remodeling to inferior fronto-parietal regions. *Brain Structure and Function*, *220*(4), 2315–2331. doi:10.1007/500429-04-0789-6

Henshilwood, C., & Dubreuil, B. (2011). The Still Bay and Howiesons Poort, 77–59: Symbolic culture and the evolution of the mind during the African middle stone age. *Current Anthropology*, *52*(3), 361–400.

Herzlinger, G., Wynn, T., & Goren-Inbar, N. (2017). Expert cognition in the production sequence of Acheulian cleavers at Gesher Benot Ya-aqov, Israel: A lithic and cognitive analysis. *PLoS One*, *12*(11), e0188337.

Hodgson, D. (2000). Art, perception and information processing: An evolutionary perspective. *Rock Art Research*, *17*, 3–34.

Hodgson, D. (2006). Understanding the origins of paleoart: The neurovisual resonance theory and brain functioning. *PaleoAnthroology*, 54–67.

Hodgson, D. (2009). Evolution of the visual cortex and the emergence of symmetry in the Acheulean techno-complex. *Comptes Rendus Palevol*, *8*, 93–97.

Hodgson, D. (2014). Decoding the Blombos engravings, shell beads and Diepkloof ostrich eggshell patterns. *Cambridge Archaeological Journal*, *24*(1), 57–69.

Hodgson, D. (2015). The symmetry of Acheulean handaxes and cognitive evolution. *Journal of Archaeological Science: Reports*, *2*, 204–208.

Hodgson, D. (2017). Deciphering patterns in the archaeology of South Africa: The neurovisual resonance theory. In T. Wynn & F. L. Coolidge (Eds.), *Cognitive models in palaeolithic archaeology* (pp. 133–156). Oxford University Press.

Holloway, R. (1969). Culture: A human domain. *Current Anthropology*, *10*, 395–412.

Houser, N., & Kloesel, C. (Eds.). (1992). *The essential peirce*. Indiana University Press.

Hovers, E. (2012). Invention, reinvention and innovation: The makings of Oldowan lithic technology. *Developments in Quaternary Science*, *16*, 51–68.

Humphrey, N. (1976). The social function of intellect. In P. Bateson & R. Hinde (Eds.), *Growing points in ethology*. Cambridge University Press.

Isaac, G. (1976). Stages of cultural elaboration in the Pleistocene: Possible archaeological indicators of the development of language capabilities. In S. Harnad, H. Steklis, & J. Lancaster (Eds.), *Origins and evolution of language and speech* (Vol. Annals 280, pp. 275–288). New York Academy of Science.

Jolly, A. (1985). *The evolution of primate behavior* (2nd ed.). Macmillan.

Kandel, E. R. (2009). The biology of memory: A forty-year perspective. *Journal of Neuroscience*, *29*(41), 12748–12756.

Keller, C., & Keller, J. (1996). *Cognition and tool use: The blacksmith at work*. Cambridge University Press.

Kellogg, R. (1969). *Analyzing children's art*. National Press Books.

Key, A., & Lycett, J. (2017). Influence of handaxe size and shape on cutting efficiency: A large-scale experiment and morphometric analysis. *Journal of Archaeological Method and Theory*, *24*, 514–541.

Knight, C. (2006). *Language, Ochre and the rule of law*. Paper presented at the Cradle of Language Conference, Stellenbosch, South Africa.

Knott, C. (2001). Female reproductive ecology of the apes: Implications for human evolution. In P. Ellison (Ed.), *Reproductive ecology and human evolution* (pp. 429–462). Aldine.

Kohn, M., & Mithen, S. (1999). Handaxes: Products of sexual selection? *Antiquity*, *73*, 518–526.

Kuhn, T. (1962). *The structure of scientific revolutions*. University of Chicago Press.

Lakoff, G., & Johnson, M. (1980). *Metaphors we live by*. University of Chicago Press.

Lakoff, G., & Johnson, M. (1999). *Philosophy in the flesh: The embodied mind and its challenge to western thought*. Basic Books.

Leakey, L. S. B. (1931). *The stone age cultures of Kenya Colony*. Cambridge University Press.

Leder, H., Belke, B., Oeberst, A., & Augustin, D. (2004). A model of aesthetic appreciation and aesthetic judgments. *British Journal of Psychology*, *95*, 489–508.

Leder, H., & Nadal, M. (2014). Ten years of a model of aesthetic appreciation and aesthetic judgments: The aesthetic episode—developments and challenges in empirical aesthetics. *British Journal of Psychology*, *105*, 443–464.

Liu, Y., Lu, X., Wu, F., Shen, M., & Gao, Z. (2019). Biological motion is stored independently from bound representation in working memory. *Visual Cognition*, *27*(9–10). doi:10.1080/13506285.2019.1638479

Lombard, M., & Haidle, M. (2012). Thinking a bow-and-arrow set: Cognitive implications of Middle Stone Age bow and stone-tipped arrow technology. *Cambridge Archaeological Journal*, *22*, 237–264.

Lombard, M., Högberg, A., & Haidle, M. (2018). Cognition: From capuchin rock pounding to Lomekwian flake production. *Cambridge Archaeological Journal*, *29*(2), 201–231.

Lombard, M., Högberg, A., & Haidle, M. (2019). Cognition: From capuchin rock pounding to Lomekwian flake production. *Cambridge Archaeological Journal*, *29*(2), 201–231.

Luria, A. R. (1966). *Higher cortical function in man*. Basic Books.

Luria, A. R. (1973). *The working brain: An introduction to neuropsychology*. Basic Books.

Maguire, E., Gadlan, D., Johnsrude, I., Good, C., Ashburner, J., Frackowiak, R., & Frith, C. (2000). Noavigation-related structural change in hippocampi of taxi drivers. *Proceedings of the National Academy of Sciences*, *97*(8), 4398–4403.

Malafouris, L. (2008). Beads for a plastic mind: The "Blind Man's Stick" (BMS) hypothesis and the active nature of material culture. *Cambridge Archaeological Journal*, *18*(3), 401–414.

Malafouris, L. (2013). *How things shape the mind: A theory of material engagement*. MIT Press.

Malafouris, L. (2021). How does thinking relate to tool making? *Adaptive Behavior*, *29*(2), 107–121.

Mandler, J. (2004). A synopsis of the foundations of mind: Origins of conceptual thought. *Developmental Science*, *7*(5), 499–505.

Marshack, A. (1991). The Tai Plaque and calendrical notation in the upper Palaeolithic. *Cambridge Archaeological Journal*, *1*(1), 25–61.

Matsuzawa, T. (Ed.). (2001). *Primate origins of human cognition and behavior*. Springer-Verlag.

Matsuzawa, T., Humle, T., & Sugiyama, Y. (Eds.). (2011). *The chimpanzees of Bossou and Nimba*. Springer.

McPherron, S. P. (2000). Handaxes as a measure of the mental abilities of early hominids. *Journal of Archaeological Science*, *27*, 655–663.

Miller, G. (1956). The magical number seven, plus or minus two: Some limits of our capacity for processing information. *Psychological Review*, 63, 81–97.

Moore, M. (2011). The design space of stone flaking: Implications for cognitive evolution. *World Archaeology*, *43*(4), 702–715.

Moore, M., & Perston, Y. (2016). Experimental insights into the cognitive significance of early stone tools. *PLoS One*, *11*(7). doi:10.1371/journal.pone.0158803

Mora, R., & de la Torre, I. (2005). Percussion tools in Olduvai Beds I and II (Tanzania): Implications for early human activities. *Journal of Anthropological Archaeology*, *24*, 179–192.

Morgan, T. J. H., Uomini, N., Rendell, L. E., Chouinard-Thuly, L., Street, S. E., Lewis, H., Cross, C. P., Evans, C., Kearney, R., de la Torre, I., Whiten, A., & Laland, K. N. (2015). Experimental evidence for the co-evolution of hominin tool-making teaching and language. *Nature Communications*, 6, 6029. doi:10.1038/ncomms7029

Niţul, E. C., Ca^rciumaru, M., Micolae, A., Cı^rstina, O., Lupu, F., & Leu, M. (2019). Mobility and social identity in the mid upper Paleolithic: New personal ornaments from Poiana Cireşului (Piatra Neamţ, Romania). *PLoS One*. doi:10.1371/journal.pone.0214932

Orban, G., & Caruana, F. (2014). The neural basis of human tool use. *Frontiers in Psychology*, 5, Article 310. doi:10.3389/fpsyg.2014.00310

Orban, G., Claeys, K., Nelissen, K., Smans, R., Sunaert, S., Todd, J., Wardak, C., Durand J. B., & Vanduffel, W. (2006). Mapping the parietal cortex of human and non-human primates. *Neuropsychologia*, *44*, 2647–2667.

Osiurak, F., Lesourd, M., Navarro, J., & Reynaud, E. (2020). Technition: When tools come out of the closet. *Perspectives on Psychological Science*, *15*(4), 880–897.

Osiurak, F., & Reynaud, E. (2020). The elephant in the China shop: When technical reasoning meets cumulative technological culture. *Behavioral and Brain Sciences*, 43.

Overmann, K. (2013). Material scaffolds in numbers and time. *Cambridge Archaeological Journal*, *23*, 19–39.

Overmann, K. (2016). The role of materiality in numerical cognition. *Quaternary International*, 405, 42–51

Overmann, K. (2017). Materiality and numerical cognition: A material engagement theory perspective. In T. Wynn & F. Coolidge (Eds.), *Cognitive models in palaeolithic archaeology* (pp. 89–112). Oxford: Oxford University Press.

Overmann, K. (2021). The material difference in human cognition. *Adaptive Behavior*, *29*(2), 123–135.

Pargeter, J., Khreisheh, N., & Stout, D. (2019). Understanding stone tool-making skill acquisition: Experimental methods and evolutionary implications. *Journal of Human Evolution*, *133*, 146–166.

Parker, S., & Gibson, K. (1979). A developmental model for the evolution of language and intelligence in early hominids. *Behavioral and Brain Sciences*, *2*, 367–408.

Parker Pearson, M. (2012). *Stonehenge: Exploring the greatest stone age mystery*. Simon & Schuster.

Pettitt, P. (2013). *The palaeolithic origins of human burial*. Routledge.

Piaget, J. (1960). *The psychology of intelligence*. Littlefield, Adams.

Piaget, J. (1970). *Genetic epistemology* (E. Duckworth, Trans.). Viking.

Piaget, J., & Inhelder, B. (1967). *The child's conception of space* (F. Langlon & J. Lunzer, Trans.). Norton.

Povenelli, D. (1987). Monkeys, apes, mirrors and minds: The evolution of self-awareness in primates. *Human Evolution*, *2*(6), 493–509.

Putt, S., Woods, A., & Franciscus, R. (2014). The role of verbal interaction during experimental bifacial stone tool manufacture. *Lithic Technology*, *39*, 96–112.

Ramachandran, V., & Hirstein, W. (1999). The science of art: A neurological theory of aesthetic experience. *Journal of Consciousness Studies*, *6*(6–7), 15–51.

Robb, J. E. (1998). The archaeology of symbols. *Annual Review of Anthropology*, *27*(1), 329–346.

Roberts, M. A., & Parfitt, S. A. (1999). *Boxgrove: A middle pleistocene hominid site at Eartham Quarry, Boxgrove, West Sussex*. English Heritage.

Roche, H., & Texier, P. (1995). Evaluation of technical competence of *Homo erectus* in East Africa during the middle Pleistocene. In J. Bower & S. Sartono (Eds.), *Evolution and ecology of Homo erectus* (pp. 153–167). Pithecanthropus Centennial Foundation.

Roebroeks, W. (1988). *From find scatters to early hominid behaviour: A study of middle palaeolithic riverside settlements at Maastricht-Belvedere (The Netherlands)* (Vol. 21). University of Leiden.

Rubin, D. C. (Ed.). (1999). *Remembering our past: Studies in autobiographical memory*. Cambridge University Press.

Sackett, J. (1982). Approaches to style in lithic archaeology. *Journal of Anthropological Archaeology*, *1*, 59–112.

Schacter, D. L. (2012). Adaptive constructive processes and the future of memory. *American Psychologist*, *67*(8), 603–613.

Schacter, D. L., & Addis, D. R. (2007). The cognitive neuroscience of constructive memory: Remembering the past and imagining the future. *Philosophical Transactions of the Royal Society B: Biological Sciences*, *362*(1481), 773–786.

Schacter, D. L., Guerin, S. A., & Jacques, P. L. S. (2011). Memory distortion: An adaptive perspective. *Trends in Cognitive Sciences*, *15*(10), 467–474.

Schlanger, N. (1996). Understanding Levallois: Lithic technology and cognitive archaeology. *Cambridge Archaeological Journal*, *6*(2), 231–254.

Semaw, S. (2000). The world's oldest stone artefacts from Gona, Ethiopia: Their implications for understanding stone technology and patterns of human evolution between 2.6–1.5 million years ago. *Journal of Archaeological Science*, *27*, 1197–1214.

Semaw, S., Rogers, M., & Stout, D. (2009). Insights into late Pliocene lithic assemblage variability: The East Gona and Ounda Gona South Oldowan archaeology (2.6 million years ago), Afar, Ethiopia. In K. Schick & N. Toth (Eds.), *The cutting edge: New approaches to the archaeology of human origins* (pp. 211–246). Stone Age Institute Press.

Shea, J., & Sisk, M. (2010). Complex projectile technology and *Homo sapiens* dispersal into Western Eurasia. *PaleoAnthropology*, *2010*, 100–122.

Shepard, R. N. (1997). The genetic basis of human scientific knowledge. In G. R. Bock & G. Cardew (Eds.), *Characterizing human psychological adaptations* (pp. 4–13). Wiley & Sons.

Shipton, C., & White, M. (2020). Handaxe types, colonization waves, and social norms in the British Acheulean. *Journal of Archaeological Science: Reports*, *31*, Article 102352.

Silverman, I., Choi, J., Mackewn, A., Fisher, M., Moro, J., & Olshansky, E. (2000). Evolved mechanisms underlying wayfinding: Further studies on the hunter-gatherer theory of spatial sex differences. *Evolution and Human Behavior*, *21*, 201–213.

Silverman, I., Choi, J., & Peters, M. (2007). The hunter-gatherer theory of sex differences in spatial abilities: Data from 40 countries. *Archives of Sexual Behavior*, *36*, 261–268.

Squire, L. R. (2004). Memory systems of the brain: A brief history and current perspective. *Neurobiology of Learning and Memory*, *82*(3), 171–177.

Stout, D., & Chaminade, T. (2007). The evolutionary neuroscience of tool making. *Neuropsychologia*, *45*, 1091–1100.

Stout, D., & Chaminade, T. (2012). Stone tools, language and the brain in human evolution. *Philosophical Transactions of the Royal Society of London, B, 367*, 75–87.

Stout, D., & Hecht, E. (2017). Evolutionary neuroscience of cumulative culture. *Proceedings of the National Academy of Sciences, 114*(30), 7861–7868. doi:10.1073/pnas.1620738114

Stout, D., Hecht, E., Khreisheh, N., Bradley, B., & Chaminade, T. (2015). Cognitive demands of lower Palaeolithic toolmaking. *PLoS One, 10*(4).

Stout, D., Schick, K., & Toth, N. (2009). Understanding Oldowan knapping skill: An experimental study of skill acquisition in modern humans. In K. Schick & N. Toth (Eds.), *The cutting edge: New approaches to the archaeology of human origins* (pp. 247–266). Stone Age Institute Press.

Stout, D., Toth, N., Schick, K., Stout, J., & Hutchins, G. (2000). Stone tool-making and brain activation: Positron emission tomography (PET) studies. *Journal of Archaeological Science, 27*, 1215–1223.

Svoboda, J. (2020). *Dolni vestonica-pavlov: Explaining paleolithic settlements in Central Europe*. Texas A&M Press.

Tennie, C., Premo, L. S., Braun, D., & McPherron, A. (2017). Early stone tools and cultural transmission: Resetting the null hypothesis. *Current Anthropology, 58*(5), 652–672.

Tomasello, M., & Call, J. (1997). *Primate cognition*. Oxford University Press.

Tomasello, M., & Herrmann, E. (2010). Ape and human cognition: What's the difference? *Current Directions in Psychological Science, 19*(1), 3–8.

Toth, N. (1987). Behavioral inferences from early stone age artifact assemblages: An experimental model. *Journal of Human Evolution, 16*, 763–787.

Toth, N., & Schick, K. (1986). The first million years: The archaeology of protohuman culture. In M. Schiffer (Ed.), *Advances in archaeological method and theory* (Vol. 9, pp. 1–96). Academic Press.

Toth, N., & Schick, K. (2018). An overview of the cognitive implications of the Oldowan industrial complex. *Azania: Archaeological Research in Africa, 53*(1), 3–39.

Toth, N., Schick, K., Savage-Rumbaugh, S., Sevcik, R., & Rumbaugh, D. (1993). *Pan* the tool-maker: Investigations into the stone tool-making and tool-using capabilities of a bonobo (*Pan paniscus*). *Journal of Archaeological Science, 20*, 81–91.

Toth, N., Schick, K., & Semaw, S. (2006). A comparative study of the stone tool-making skills of *Pan*, *Australopithecus*, and *Homo sapiens*. In N. Toth & K. Schick (Eds.), *The oldowan: Case studies into the earliest stone age* (pp. 155–222). Stone Age Institute Press.

Trinkaus, E., & Buzhilova, A. (2018). Diversity and differential disposal of the dead at Sunghir. *Antiquity, 92*(361), 7–21.

Tulving, E. (1995). Organization of memory: Quo vadis? In M. S. Gazzaniga (Ed.), *The cognitive neurosciences* (pp. 839–853). The MIT Press.

Twomey, T. (2013). The cognitive implications of controlled use of fire. *Cambridge Archaeological Journal, 23*(1), 113–128.

Wadley, L. (2010). Were snares and traps used in the middle stone age and does it matter? A review and a case study from Sibudu, South Africa. *Journal of Human Evolution, 58*(2), 179–192.

Wadley, L., Hodgskiss, T., & Grant, M. (2009). Hafting tools with compound adhesives in the middle stone age, South Africa: Implications for complex cognition. *Proceedings of the National Academy of Sciences, 106*, 9590–9594.

Walker, M., Anesin, D., Angelucci, D., Aviles-Fernandez, A., Buitrago-Lopez, A., Fernandez-Jalvo, Y., Haber-Uriarte, M., López-Jiménez, A., López-Martínez, M.,

Martín-Lerma, I., Ortega-Rodrigáñez, J., Polo-Camacho, J. L., Rhodes, S. E., Richter, D., Rodríguez-Estrella, T., Schwenninger, J. L., & Skinner, A. (2016). Combustion at the late early Pleistocene site of Cueva Negra de Estrecho del Rio Quipar (Murcia, Spain). *Antiquity*, *90*(351), 571–589.

Weber, B., & Depew, D. (Eds.). (2003). *Evolution and learning: The baldwin effect reconsidered*. MIT Press.

Whiten, A., Schick, K., & Toth, N. (2009). The evolution and cultural transmission of percussive technology: Integrating evidence from palaeoanthrology and primatology. *Journal of Human Evolution*, *57*, 420–435.

Whitley, D. S. (2008). Archaeological evidence for conceptual metaphors as enduring knowledge structures. *Time and Mind: The Journal of Archaeology, Consciousness, and Culture*, *1*(1), 7–29.

Whittle, A. (1996). *Europe in the neolithic: The creation of new worlds*. Cambridge University Press.

Winograd, E., & Neisser, U. (Eds.). (2006). *Affect and accuracy in recall: Studies of "Flashbulb" memories* (Vol. 4). Cambridge University Press.

Wrangham, R. W. (2009). *Catching fire: How cooking made us human*. Basic Books.

Wynn, R., & Coolidge, F. (2009). Does greater phonological storage capacity correlate with levels of intentionality and theory of mind? *Psychological Reports*, *105*, 625–632.

Wynn, T. (1979). The intelligence of later Acheulean hominids. *Man*, *14*, 371–391.

Wynn, T. (1989). *The evolution of spatial competence*. University of Illinois Press.

Wynn, T. (1991). Tools, grammar, and the archaeology of cognition. *Cambridge Archaeological Journal*, *1*, 191–206.

Wynn, T. (2002). Archaeology and cognitive evolution. *Behavioral and Brain Sciences*, *25*(3), 389–438.

Wynn, T. (2009). Hafted spears and the archaeology of mind. *Proceedings of the National Academy of Sciences*, *106*(24), 9544–9545.

Wynn, T. (2010). The evolution of human spatial cognition. In F. Dolins (Ed.), *Spatial perception, spatial cognition* (pp. 213–236). Cambridge University Press.

Wynn, T. (2021). Ergonomic clusters and displaced affordances in early lithic technology. *Adaptive Behavior*, *29*(2), 181–195.

Wynn, T., & Berlant, T. (2019). The handaxe aesthetic. In K. Overmann & F. Coolidge (Eds.), *Squeezing minds from stones: Cognitive archaeology and the evolution of the human mind* (pp. 278–303). Oxford University Press.

Wynn, T., & Coolidge, F. (2009). Implications of a strict standard for recognizing modern cognition in prehistory. In S. De Baune, F. Coolidge, & T. Wynn (Eds.), *Cognitive archaeology and human evolution* (pp. 117–127). Cambridge University Press.

Wynn, T., & Coolidge, F. L. (2010a). How Levallois reduction is similar to, and not similar to, playing chess. In A. Nowell & I. Davidson (Eds.), *Stone tools and the evolution of human cognition* (pp. 83–104). University of Colorado Press.

Wynn, T., & Coolidge, F. L. (Eds.). (2010b). Working memory: Beyond language and symbolism. *Current Anthropology*, *51* (Supplement 1).

Wynn, T., & Coolidge, F. (2012). *How to think like a neandertal*. Oxford University Press.

Wynn, T., & Coolidge, F. (2014). Technical cognition, working memory, and creativity. *Pragmatics and Cognition*, *22*(1), 45–63.

Wynn, T., & Coolidge, F. (2016). Archaeological insights into hominin cognitive evolution. *Evolutionary Anthropology*, *25*, 200–213. doi:10.002/evan.21496

Wynn, T., Coolidge, F., & Bright, M. (2009). Hohlenstein-Stadel and the evolution of human conceptual thought. *Cambridge Archaeological Journal*, *19*(1), 73–83.

Wynn, T., Haidle, M., Lombard, M., & Coolidge, F. (2017). The expert cognition model in human evolutionary studies. In T. Wynn & F. Coolidge (Eds.), *Cognitive models in palaeolithic archaeology* (pp. 21–44). Oxford University Press.

Wynn, T., Overmann, K., & Coolidge, F. (2016). The false dichotomy: A refutation of the Neandertal indistinguishability claim. *Journal of Anthropological Sciences*, *94*, 1–22.

Wynn, T., Overmann, K., Coolidge, F., & Janulis, K. (2017). Bootstrapping ordinal thinking. In T. Wynn & F. Coolidge (Eds.), *Cognitive models in palaeolithic archaeology* (pp. 197–213). Oxford University Press.

Wynn, T., Sahnouni, M., Berlant, T., & Douce, C. (2020). Reflections on possible zoomorphic Acheulean bifaces from southwestern Algeria. In J. Cole, J. McNabb, M. Grove, & R. Hosfield (Eds.), *Landscapes of evolution: Contributions in honour of John Gowlett* (pp. 117–124). Archaeopress.

Zeki, S. (1999). *Inner vision: An exploration of art and the brain*. Oxford University Press.

Zilhao, J., Angelucci, D., Badal-Garcia, E., d'Errico, F., Daniel, F., Dayet, L., Douka, K., Higham, T. F. G., Martínez-Sánchez, M. J., Montes-Bernárdez, R., Murcia-Mascarós, S., Pérez-Sirvent, C., Roldán-García, C., Vanhaeren, M., Villaverde, V., Wood, R., Zapata, J., & Zapata, J. (2010). Symbolic use of marine shells and mineral pigments by Iberian Neandertals. *Proceedings of the National Academy of Sciences*, *107*(3), 1023–1028.

Index

www.ingramcontent.com/pod-product-compliance
Ingram Content Group UK Ltd.
Pitfield, Milton Keynes, MK11 3LW, UK
UKHW022018180926
475701UK00005B/909
* 9 7 8 0 3 6 7 8 5 6 9 4 6 *